Current Topics in Emerging and Reemerging Zoonoses

Edited by Alfonso J. Rodriguez-Morales

Published in London, United Kingdom

Current Topics in Emerging and Reemerging Zoonoses
http://dx.doi.org/10.5772/intechopen.1006230
Edited by Alfonso J. Rodriguez-Morales

Contributors
Alfonso J. Rodriguez-Morales, Aliya Rizvi, Daniel Nunez-Avellaneda, Danish Nasar Khan, Eman S. Elwakil, Gayatree Nayak, Haleema H. Albohiri, Henry Puerta-Guardo, Jeebanjyoti Mishra, Luis Antonio Alonso-Palomares, Maneesh Kumar, Manuel Alejandro Mosso Pani, Mithilesh Kumar Jha, Monalisa Mohanty, Muslimah N. Alsulami, Nicole M. Nazario Maldonado, Pratima Gupta, Preetam Kumar Kar, Ratnesh Kumar, Sarah Albalawi, Suman Kumar, Sutapa Rath

First published in London, United Kingdom, 2025 by IntechOpen
IntechOpen is the global imprint of INTECHOPEN LIMITED, registered in England and Wales, registration number: 11086078, 167-169 Great Portland Street, London, W1W 5PF, United Kingdom

For EU product safety concerns: IN TECH d.o.o., Prolaz Marije Krucifikse Kozulić 3, 51000 Rijeka, Croatia, info@intechopen.com or visit our website at intechopen.com.

British Library Cataloguing-in-Publication Data
A catalogue record for this book is available from the British Library

Current Topics in Emerging and Reemerging Zoonoses
Edited by Alfonso J. Rodriguez-Morales
p. cm.
Print ISBN 978-1-83635-256-3
Online ISBN 978-1-83635-255-6
eBook (PDF) ISBN 978-1-83635-257-0

Meet the editor

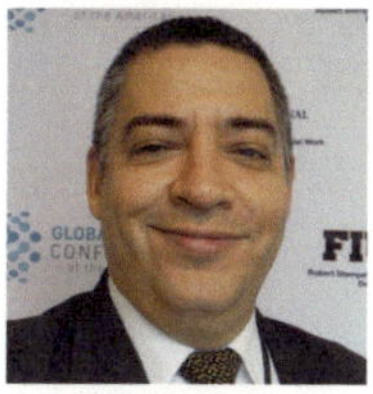

Dr. Alfonso J. Rodriguez-Morales received his MD from Universidad Central de Venezuela in Caracas and his MSc in Protozoology/Parasitology from Universidad de Los Andes in Trujillo, Venezuela. He received his Diploma in Tropical Medicine & Hygiene (DTM&H) from Universidad Peruana Cayetano Heredia, Lima, Peru, and the University of Alabama at Birmingham, Alabama, USA. He also holds a DipEd. Dr. Rodriguez-Morales is a fellow of the Royal Society for Tropical Medicine & Hygiene (FRSTMH), London, United Kingdom; of the Faculty of Travel Medicine (FFTM) of the Royal College of Physicians and Surgeons of Glasgow (RCPSG), Glasgow, Scotland, United Kingdom; of the American College of Epidemiology (FACE), USA; and the International Society for Antimicrobial Chemotherapy (FISAC). He has an HonDSc from Universidad Privada Franz Tamayo (UniFranz), Cochabamba, Bolivia. He is the President of the Latin American Society for Travel Medicine (SLAMVI) (2023-2025), and the Past President of the Colombian Infectious Diseases Association (2021–2023). He is a member of the Council (2020-2026) of the International Society for Infectious Diseases (ISID). He is a senior researcher at Colciencias (2015–2027) and a professor at the Fundación Universitaria Autónoma de las Américas in Pereira, Risaralda, Colombia, as well as at the Universidad Científica del Sur (UCSUR) in Lima, Peru. He is a visiting professor at multiple national and international universities.

Contents

Preface

Emerging and reemerging zoonoses continue to represent one of the most pressing challenges to global health, security, and sustainable development. Diseases that pass from animals to humans, whether viral, bacterial, parasitic, or fungal, have repeatedly disrupted societies, economies, and healthcare systems worldwide. In recent decades, we have witnessed the steady rise and resurgence of zoonotic threats such as Ebola, avian influenza, SARS-CoV-2, mpox, Rift Valley fever, and new rickettsial infections. These events reveal the complexity of pathogen dynamics at the interface of humans, animals, and the environment, highlighting the urgent need for integrated approaches to prevention and control.

Current Topics in Emerging and Reemerging Zoonoses brings together experts from multiple fields to explore the drivers, mechanisms, and consequences of zoonotic diseases in the twenty-first century. This volume integrates perspectives from epidemiology, veterinary medicine, clinical practice, microbiology, ecology, and One Health, while also considering the social, economic, cultural, and political factors that shape zoonotic risks. It examines both long-recognized zoonoses that continue to reappear in new contexts and novel pathogens that test the limits of our preparedness.

In addition to reviewing the current body of scientific knowledge, this book emphasizes the practical implications of zoonotic research. It discusses how to improve surveillance, expand laboratory capacity, strengthen interdisciplinary collaboration, and translate findings into policies and interventions at local, national, and global levels. In a world where ecological disruption, climate change, and human mobility accelerate the emergence of new pathogens, such insights are essential for building resilient systems capable of anticipating and mitigating future crises.

We hope this volume will serve as a valuable resource for researchers, clinicians, veterinarians, and public health professionals, while also inspiring students, policymakers, and other stakeholders to participate in the shared responsibility of addressing zoonotic threats. By learning from past experiences and engaging with current challenges, we can strengthen our ability to respond to future zoonotic outbreaks and reduce their impact on both human and animal health.

Considering these issues, this book presents research and clinical topics related to what has been learned about reemerging and emerging zoonoses. The book's six chapters are organized in two major sections: "Epidemiology" and "Clinical Aspects, Diagnostics and Miscellaneous".

Commissioning this book by IntechOpen is partly related to my long commitment to tropical and emerging diseases, mainly vector-borne, zoonotic, and neglected tropical diseases. I am a member of the Council of the International Society for Infectious Diseases (ISID) (2020-2026), and Past President of the Colombian Association of Infectious Diseases (Asociación Colombiana de Infectología, ACIN) (2021-2023), as well as of the Committee on Tropical Medicine, Zoonoses and Travel Medicine of the ACIN. During 2020, I founded the Latin American Network of Research on COVID-19 (LANCOVID). LANCOVID has contributed to the research on SARS-CoV-2/COVID-19 in Latin America. Since 2024, I have been a member of the World Health Organization (WHO) Guideline Development Group for the Clinical Management of Post-COVID-19 Conditions (2024-2025) and a Member of the Expert Panel for Developing the Rapid Guideline on Mpox of the European Society for Clinical Microbiology and Infectious Diseases (ESCMID).

Following the same philosophy we used for my ten previous books with IntechOpen, this book is not intended to be an exhaustive compilation. Research on reemerging and emerging zoonoses has become highly dynamic and rapidly evolving, necessitating consultation with the most recent available evidence for informed diagnostic and treatment decisions.

I want to extend my heartfelt gratitude to IntechOpen, particularly Elvira Baumgartner, Publishing Process Manager, for entrusting me with the opportunity to edit this essential and engaging book. Her unwavering support throughout the process has been truly invaluable.

I also wish to take this moment to dedicate this book to my beloved family, who are geographically spread across Venezuela, Chile, and Colombia. Though physically apart, they remain ever close in heart. Aurora, Alfonso José, Alejandro, and Andrea (the neurologist), each of you holds a special place in my life. My deepest love and appreciation go to my wife, Katterine, my heart, my soul, and my most significant source of passion. She enriches my life every day, attentively supporting every facet of it. More than just a partner and travel companion, she is my steadfast ally in life's journey. I am deeply grateful for her presence, along with our cherished canine companions, Antonieta and Jazz. With every passing day, my love for her only grows stronger.

I am also sincerely thankful to my friends, as well as my undergraduate and postgraduate students across Colombia, Venezuela, and Latin America. Since joining the Fundación Universitaria Autónoma de las Américas in Pereira, Risaralda, Colombia, in 2019, I have found a new academic "home" that has welcomed and supported my pursuits in research and education. Special thanks are due to Dr. Maria Monica Murillo, Dean of the Faculty of Medicine, and to Dr. Jaime Cardona-Ospina, former Director of the School of Medicine, a dear friend and colleague who is now pursuing his PhD in the United States. I am equally grateful for the enduring support of Dr. José Antonio Suárez ("Tony") from Venezuela and Panama, as well as my esteemed friend, Dr. Alberto Paniz-Mondolfi, from Venezuela and the United States.

Finally, I hope our readers enjoy this book as much as I enjoyed working on it with my talented and knowledgeable collaborators.

Prof. Alfonso J. Rodriguez-Morales
MD, MSc, DTM&H, DipEd, FRSTMH(Lon), FFTM RCPS(Glasg),
FACE, FISAC, HonDSc,
Professor,
Senior Researcher, Grupo de Investigación Biomedicina,
Faculty of Medicine,
Fundación Universitaria Autónoma de las Américas – Institución
Universitaria Visión de las Américas,
Pereira, Risaralda, Colombia

Lecturer,
Universidad Científica del Sur,
Lima, Peru

President,
Latin American Society for Travel Medicine (SLAMVI),
Member of the Committee on Tropical Medicine, Zoonoses and Travel Medicine,
Colombian Association of Infectious Diseases (ACIN),
San Juan, Puerto Rico

Section 1

Epidemiology

Chapter 1

Introductory Chapter: Emerging and Reemerging Zoonoses – A Challenge in the Post-Pandemic World

Alfonso J. Rodriguez-Morales

1. Introduction

Emerging and reemerging zoonoses continue to rank among the most formidable health challenges of the twenty-first century [1]. More than 60% of human infectious diseases are zoonotic in origin, and nearly three-quarters of emerging pathogens originate from animals, underscoring the pivotal role of the human-animal-environment interface in disease ecology [2]. Whether through the reappearance of classical infections such as rabies, plague, and anthrax in specific regions, or through the global spread of novel viral threats like avian influenza, Nipah virus, and most recently SARS-CoV-2 (severe acute respiratory syndrome coronavirus 2) and monkeypox (Mpox) [3–5], zoonotic pathogens have repeatedly demonstrated their potential to destabilize health systems, disrupt economies, and challenge societies at every level [6]. The growing pace and diversity of these events underscore the urgent need for comprehensive strategies to predict, prevent, and control them [7].

Several interrelated drivers are fueling the emergence and recurrence of zoonotic diseases. Expanding globalization, deforestation, intensive agricultural practices, and climate change are reshaping ecosystems and facilitating greater contact between humans and wildlife reservoirs [8–10]. Urban expansion into previously undisturbed environments and the international wildlife trade further increase opportunities for spillover. At the same time, modern transportation networks allow outbreaks that begin locally to spread with remarkable speed across regions and continents. The coronavirus disease (COVID-19) crisis starkly illustrated these dynamics but was hardly unique; the persistence of Ebola in parts of Africa [11–20], the recent reemergence of Mpox across continents, and recurrent epidemics of arboviruses such as dengue, chikungunya, and Zika all serve as reminders that zoonoses remain both persistent and unpredictable threats [21–23].

The post-pandemic landscape has revealed both advances and weaknesses in our ability to respond to zoonotic crises. The rapid development of diagnostics and vaccines against SARS-CoV-2 showcased the potential of scientific innovation [24–30]. Yet, at the same time, inequitable access to these tools, widespread misinformation, and fragile health infrastructures hindered practical control efforts. Comparable gaps can be seen in the management of other zoonotic diseases, where insufficient surveillance, chronic underinvestment in veterinary and public health services, and limited international coordination have constrained preparedness and response. Compounding these barriers are challenges, such as political instability, social inequities, and insufficient interdisciplinary collaboration, all of which intensify the risks associated with zoonotic outbreaks [31–34].

Confronting the complexity of these threats requires a One Health framework, which acknowledges the inextricable links between human, animal, and environmental health [35–49]. Strengthening surveillance must involve not only human populations but also livestock and wildlife reservoirs. Policy frameworks should prioritize sustained collaboration across medicine, veterinary science, ecology, and the social sciences. In today's highly interconnected world, zoonoses must be recognized as more than biomedical concerns; they are equally political, economic, and cultural challenges that demand coordinated and inclusive solutions [35–51].

This volume, *Current Topics in Emerging and Reemerging Zoonoses*, brings together experts from diverse disciplines to analyze the drivers, patterns, and responses to zoonotic disease. This introductory chapter aims to contextualize the global significance of zoonoses in the post-COVID era and to emphasize the urgent need for preparedness strategies that are equitable, resilient, and multidisciplinary. History leaves little doubt that future zoonotic outbreaks are inevitable; the real challenge lies in whether humanity can learn from previous crises and transform those lessons into meaningful prevention, preparedness, and genuine global solidarity.

2. Epidemiology of emerging and reemerging zoonoses

The epidemiology of emerging and reemerging zoonoses involves analyzing their distribution, determinants, and transmission patterns across human, animal, and environmental domains. Unlike infections confined to human hosts, zoonotic diseases often originate in wildlife or domestic animals before crossing species barriers. Recognizing these patterns is essential for identifying populations at risk, anticipating spillover events, and developing preventive strategies that target both human and animal reservoirs [52, 53].

Zoonotic pathogens spread through diverse and often overlapping routes. Direct contact with infected animals or their secretions underlies diseases, such as rabies and brucellosis. In contrast, foodborne transmission from contaminated animal products is a central factor in infections like *Salmonella* and *Listeria*. Vector-borne pathogens, including those responsible for dengue, Rift Valley fever, and leishmaniasis, illustrate how arthropods can act as bridging hosts. Other zoonoses, such as avian influenza or SARS-CoV-2, may be transmitted via airborne droplets, facilitating rapid person-to-person spread once the virus adapts. Key epidemiological parameters—including the reproductive number (R_0), incubation period, duration of infectiousness, host range, and reservoir dynamics—shape the course of these outbreaks and inform control strategies [4, 23, 28, 33, 51].

Global forces are amplifying opportunities for zoonotic emergence. Deforestation, agricultural expansion, and wildlife trade increase contact between humans and potential reservoirs, while urbanization and climate variability reshape ecosystems in ways that favor vectors and pathogens. At the same time, globalization and extensive travel networks mean that localized spillover events can quickly escalate into regional or even global crises. Recent history offers stark examples: the cross-continental spread of Zika and chikungunya, recurrent Ebola epidemics in Africa, and the multi-country reemergence of Mpox [2, 9, 21, 25].

Molecular epidemiology and genomic surveillance have become indispensable for studying zoonotic outbreaks. Whole-genome sequencing provides insights into viral evolution, transmission chains, and host adaptation, allowing for near real-time monitoring of epidemic dynamics. These methods have been pivotal not only during the COVID-19 pandemic but also in tracing influenza strains circulating at the animal-human interface and investigating spillovers of Nipah, MERS (Middle East respiratory syndrome), and other coronaviruses. Nonetheless, disparities in sequencing capacity between high- and low-resource settings remain a significant barrier to equitable global monitoring [3, 4, 11, 29].

The burden of zoonotic diseases is unevenly distributed. Communities with limited healthcare access, high dependence on livestock, or proximity to wildlife are disproportionately affected. Socioeconomic inequities, cultural practices, and occupational exposures further compound vulnerability. For this reason, epidemiological studies must adopt socioecological frameworks that account for how structural and environmental determinants shape disease risk and resilience [9, 19, 43, 51, 53].

Strong surveillance systems form the cornerstone of effective zoonotic disease management. These include passive case reporting, sentinel monitoring in humans and animals, and active field surveillance of wildlife populations. Integration under a One Health paradigm, linking medical, veterinary, and ecological data, offers a more comprehensive view of risk and strengthens early warning capacity. Yet, significant obstacles persist, including resource limitations in endemic regions, fragmented data-sharing mechanisms, and geopolitical constraints [1, 2, 6, 21].

As the drivers of zoonotic emergence continue to evolve, epidemiology must adapt accordingly. Emerging approaches, such as ecological modeling, climate-informed predictive tools, and community-based participatory surveillance, can complement traditional methods. By adopting agile, inclusive, and globally coordinated strategies, the scientific and public health community can better anticipate, prevent, and mitigate the inevitable threats posed by emerging and reemerging zoonoses [19, 20, 45].

3. Main clinical impact of emerging and reemerging zoonoses

Emerging and reemerging zoonoses present complex clinical challenges that affect both patient outcomes and the resilience of health systems (**Table 1**). Since these infections often involve pathogens that originate in animals and cross into humans, their clinical manifestations can be highly variable. They range from asymptomatic or mild disease to severe and life-threatening illness. Pathogen virulence, host immune response, age, comorbidities, and access to medical care all influence the clinical spectrum. These conditions often expose critical gaps in healthcare preparedness and response [19, 37, 38, 50].

Respiratory zoonoses remain among the most consequential. Avian and swine influenza strains, together with coronaviruses of animal origin, such as SARS-CoV (severe acute respiratory syndrome coronavirus), MERS-CoV (Middle East respiratory syndrome coronavirus), and SARS-CoV-2, can cause acute respiratory syndromes with a broad range of severity. Severe cases progress to pneumonia, acute respiratory distress syndrome (ARDS), and multiple organ failure. COVID-19, in particular, demonstrated the far-reaching clinical impact of respiratory zoonoses, with complications that extended beyond the lungs to cardiovascular, neurological, and hematological systems. Prolonged

System	COVID-19 (SARS-CoV-2)	Ebola virus disease (EVD)	Zika virus	Dengue virus	Chikungunya virus	Rabies	Plague (*Yersinia pestis*)	Leptospirosis
General	Fever, fatigue, malaise	Sudden high fever, profound fatigue	Low-grade fever, rash	High fever, headache, retro-orbital pain	High fever, rash, fatigue	Prodromal fever, paresthesia	Fever, chills, malaise	Fever, chills, myalgia
Respiratory	Cough, dyspnea, hypoxia; ARDS in severe cases	Cough rare, due to systemic compromise	Mild or absent respiratory symptoms	Usually absent	Occasional mild cough	Aerophobia, hydrophobia due to spasms	Pneumonia (pneumonic plague)	Cough, pulmonary hemorrhage (severe cases)
Cardiovascular	Tachycardia, myocarditis, thromboembolism	Hypotension, shock in late stages	Rare fetal bradycardia	Hypotension, plasma leakage (severe dengue)	Rare arrhythmias, possible myocarditis	Cardiac arrhythmias (late stage)	Hypotension, septic shock (septicemic plague)	Hypotension, myocarditis (severe cases)
Neurological	Headache, anosmia, encephalopathy, stroke	Confusion, delirium, seizures (late)	Guillain-Barré syndrome, congenital Zika syndrome	Encephalopathy, seizures (rare)	Polyarthritis, neuroinflammation (rare)	Encephalitis, paralysis, coma	Meningitis (rare, meningeal plague)	Aseptic meningitis, encephalitis (rare)
Gastrointestinal (GI)	Diarrhea, nausea, vomiting	Profuse vomiting, diarrhea, abdominal pain	Nausea, vomiting occasionally	Nausea, abdominal pain, vomiting	Nausea, vomiting, mild diarrhea	Dysphagia, pharyngeal spasms	Abdominal pain, hepatosplenomegaly	Abdominal pain, nausea, jaundice
Musculoskeletal	Myalgia, fatigue	Severe myalgia, weakness	Mild arthralgia	Myalgia, arthralgia	Severe arthralgia, chronic arthritis-like symptoms	Muscle spasms, rigidity	Myalgia, tender lymph nodes (buboes)	Severe myalgia, calf tenderness
Dermatologic	Rash (infrequent), chilblain-like lesions	Petechiae, rash, bleeding in late disease	Maculopapular rash, conjunctivitis	Maculopapular rash, bleeding (severe dengue)	Maculopapular rash, facial flushing	Nonspecific (bite wound site)	Black necrotic skin lesions (bubonic plague)	Conjunctival suffusion, rash (occasionally)
Hematologic	Lymphopenia, thrombocytopenia, elevated D-dimer	Leukopenia, thrombocytopenia, liver enzyme elevation	Mild leukopenia	Thrombocytopenia, hemoconcentration	Mild thrombocytopenia, lymphopenia	Nonspecific leukocytosis	Leukocytosis, coagulopathy	Leukocytosis, thrombocytopenia
Imaging	Chest CT: ground-glass opacities, consolidation	GI imaging may show fluid accumulation	Neuroimaging: calcifications in congenital cases	Chest X-ray: pleural effusion (severe dengue)	Joint imaging: synovitis, tenosynovitis	MRI/CT: encephalitis changes (late)	Chest X-ray: infiltrates (pneumonic form)	Chest X-ray: alveolar infiltrates; renal ultrasound: nephritis

Table 1.
Main clinical, laboratory, and imaging findings of some selected reemerging and emerging zoonoses by organs and systems.

post-viral syndromes added another layer of complexity. The unprecedented demand for intensive care and ventilatory support during pandemic peaks highlighted systemic vulnerabilities in many countries [15, 20, 23, 34, 47].

Hemorrhagic zoonotic diseases are also of significant concern because of their high fatality rates. Infections such as Ebola, Marburg, Lassa fever, and Crimean-Congo hemorrhagic fever are characterized by fever, vascular leakage, coagulopathy, and progressive multiorgan dysfunction. These pathogens often emerge in regions with fragile health systems where advanced supportive care and high-level isolation are not available. Clinical outcomes are usually poor without early diagnosis and immediate intervention, emphasizing the need for rapid recognition and effective supportive therapy [54–57].

Arboviral zoonoses, such as dengue, chikungunya, Zika, and yellow fever, illustrate the broad clinical spectrum of vector-borne diseases [58–72]. Dengue can manifest as a mild febrile illness or evolve into severe hemorrhagic fever and shock. Zika virus, often mild in adults, is linked to congenital Zika syndrome, which includes microcephaly and other neurodevelopmental disorders. Chikungunya is mainly associated with febrile polyarthritis that may persist chronically and significantly affect quality of life. Yellow fever continues to cause acute hepatitis, renal impairment, and hemorrhagic complications that can be fatal without adequate care [73–84].

Neurotropic zoonotic viruses are another vital source of morbidity and mortality. Rabies, Japanese encephalitis, and West Nile virus can invade the central nervous system, leading to encephalitis, meningitis, or paralytic syndromes. Rabies remains almost universally fatal, once symptoms appear. Japanese encephalitis and West Nile virus can result in long-term neurological impairment, particularly in children, older adults, and immunocompromised individuals [85–87].

The clinical impact of zoonoses often persists well beyond the acute stage of illness. Sequelae involving the nervous, cardiovascular, renal, and psychiatric systems are increasingly recognized. Health services face the dual burden of managing acutely ill patients while also providing rehabilitation and long-term follow-up. Outbreaks exert a psychological toll on patients and healthcare workers alike, with stress, anxiety, and burnout being common consequences that are frequently underestimated [16, 27, 44, 86, 87].

Coinfections complicate clinical management. In endemic regions, patients are often simultaneously exposed to zoonotic diseases and conditions, such as malaria, HIV (human immunodeficiency virus), or tuberculosis. These interactions can worsen severity, obscure diagnosis, and alter therapeutic responses. Immunocompromised individuals are at particular risk of atypical presentations, prolonged viral shedding, and poor outcomes [54, 60, 63, 86].

The lack of specific antiviral therapies remains a significant challenge in the management of many zoonotic infections. Clinical care is often limited to supportive measures, including fluid replacement, respiratory assistance, and symptomatic treatment. Vaccines provide adequate protection against some diseases, such as rabies and yellow fever, but coverage and availability remain uneven. The rapid development of COVID-19 vaccines showed the possibilities of modern biotechnology, but many other zoonotic pathogens still lack vaccines or specific treatments [1, 12, 59, 73].

4. Research challenges on emerging and reemerging zoonoses

The research landscape surrounding emerging and reemerging zoonoses is uniquely complex, shaped by the intersection of human, animal, and environmental health. As zoonotic diseases continue to cause recurrent outbreaks and global health crises, robust and timely research is essential to guide surveillance, therapeutic development, and preventive strategies. Yet, scientific investigation in this field faces significant logistical, ethical, and structural obstacles that often limit the generation of high-quality evidence [88–90].

A fundamental challenge is the unpredictability of zoonotic spillover events. Outbreaks frequently arise without warning, in settings where preapproved research protocols and rapid mobilization of resources are not in place. This delay often results in missed opportunities for data collection. For instance, investigations during successive Ebola epidemics were hindered by difficulties in launching clinical trials quickly enough to evaluate promising treatments in real time. Similar problems occur with other zoonoses, where research frameworks are typically reactive rather than anticipatory [91–93].

Infrastructure limitations also hinder research, especially in the low- and middle-income countries where many zoonotic outbreaks originate. Weak laboratory systems, insufficient diagnostic capacity, lack of trained personnel, and chronic underfunding all constrain rapid pathogen identification, genomic surveillance, and clinical research. These deficiencies contribute to delayed outbreak detection, inadequate case characterization, and fragmented data reporting [94–96].

Ethical concerns further complicate research during zoonotic outbreaks. The urgency to generate evidence must be balanced against the responsibility to safeguard vulnerable populations, ensure informed consent, and guarantee equitable access to investigational interventions. Designing and implementing randomized controlled trials during the midst of an outbreak is particularly challenging, as seen in Ebola and Lassa fever epidemics, where the humanitarian imperative to offer experimental treatments often conflicted with the requirements of scientific rigor [16, 27, 91].

Data sharing and coordination represent another persistent obstacle. Institutional barriers, proprietary restrictions, and geopolitical tensions frequently delay the dissemination of critical epidemiological and genomic data. The COVID-19 pandemic demonstrated both the value of open science and the risks of fragmented information flows. For zoonoses, where animal reservoirs and cross-border spread are common, failure to share data promptly undermines effective surveillance and control [12, 15, 34].

Finally, research funding for zoonotic diseases is often reactive and short-lived. Investment tends to surge during outbreaks but declines once the immediate crisis subsides. This cyclical funding undermines sustained progress in surveillance, vaccine development, and therapeutic innovation, leaving the world unprepared for the subsequent inevitable emergence [43, 55, 74].

Addressing these challenges requires strengthening global research collaboration and building resilient networks that bridge human, veterinary, and environmental health. Equitable funding mechanisms, adaptable ethical frameworks, and investment in laboratory and genomic capacity in endemic regions are essential. By fostering agile, inclusive, and transparent research systems, the scientific community can generate timely evidence and contribute to a more coordinated response to both current and future zoonotic threats [22, 36, 45].

5. Conclusions

Emerging and reemerging zoonoses have become an enduring challenge to global health, testing the resilience of healthcare systems, scientific capacity, and international collaboration. From rabies and plague to Ebola, avian influenza, Zika, and COVID-19, these diseases illustrate how the human-animal-environment interface continues to generate critical vulnerabilities in surveillance, clinical management, and research readiness. As emphasized in this chapter, the challenges are multidimensional, encompassing epidemiological complexity, clinical burden, scientific obstacles, and the urgent need for coordinated global action.

From an epidemiological perspective, zoonoses thrive in conditions shaped by ecological disruption, globalization, deforestation, urban expansion, and climate variability. Spillover from wildlife or livestock into human populations, compounded by modern travel and trade, allows localized events to evolve rapidly into regional or global crises. Vigilant monitoring systems and real-time data sharing are therefore indispensable. A One Health approach that integrates human, veterinary, and environmental health remains the cornerstone for anticipating and mitigating zoonotic threats.

Clinically, zoonotic diseases manifest across multiple organ systems and produce outcomes ranging from mild infection to severe multiorgan failure and death. Their burden is not limited to acute illness; long-term sequelae, disability, and psychological consequences are increasingly recognized. Moreover, social determinants of health, preexisting conditions, and inequities in healthcare access strongly influence disease outcomes. For many zoonotic pathogens, the lack of specific antivirals or effective vaccines means that early diagnosis, supportive care, and preventive strategies remain the primary pillars of management.

Research on zoonoses, while essential, is fraught with obstacles. Unpredictable outbreaks, limited infrastructure in endemic regions, ethical and logistical challenges, and inequities in funding and capacity all impede the ability to generate timely evidence. The experience of COVID-19 and repeated Ebola outbreaks has demonstrated both the potential of agile research frameworks and the persistent disparities in scientific infrastructure between countries. Open science, cross-sector collaboration, and sustained investment in laboratory and genomic capacity are vital to addressing these shortcomings.

Looking forward, the global community must transition from reactive responses to proactive preparedness. This involves investing in integrated surveillance networks, strengthening healthcare delivery and veterinary services, supporting interdisciplinary research, and ensuring equitable access to diagnostics, therapeutics, and vaccines. Building resilience requires innovation, transparency, trust, and solidarity across borders.

This chapter has laid the foundation for deeper exploration of the drivers, dynamics, and impacts of emerging and reemerging zoonoses presented in this volume. By advancing our understanding of the underlying challenges and potential responses, the aim is to contribute to a more coordinated, evidence-based, and equitable global strategy to confront zoonotic threats in the post-pandemic world.

Acknowledgements

The author acknowledges the use of Grammarly Premium® Academic, as well as PubMed, Scopus, and Web of Sciences for searching supporting articles, and Microsoft® Editor/Copilot for language polishing of the manuscript. Additionally, EndNote is used for managing references, and Microsoft Word for Windows, running on a Dell Inspiron laptop, is used for writing.

Author details

Alfonso J. Rodriguez-Morales[1,2,3,4]

1 Grupo de Investigación Biomedicina, Faculty of Medicine, Fundación Universitaria Autónoma de las Américas-Institución Universitaria Visión de las Américas, Pereira, Risaralda, Colombia

2 Universidad Cientifica del Sur, Lima, Peru

3 Latin American Society for Travel Medicine (SLAMVI), San Juan, Puerto Rico

4 Committee on Tropical Medicine, Zoonoses and Travel Medicine, Asociación Colombiana de Infectología (ACIN), Bogotá, DC, Colombia

*Address all correspondence to: ajrodriguezmmd@gmail.com

References

[1] Cardenas R, Sandoval CM, Rodriguez-Morales AJ, Vivas P. Zoonoses and climate variability. Annals of the New York Academy of Sciences. 2008;**1149**:326-330

[2] Cascio A, Pernice LM, Barberi G, Delfino D, Biondo C, Beninati C, et al. Secondary hemophagocytic lymphohistiocytosis in zoonoses. A systematic review. European Review for Medical and Pharmacological Sciences. 2012;**16**(10):1324-1337

[3] Al-Kassab-Cordova A, Ulloque-Badaracco JR, Benites-Zapata VA, Sah R, Rodriguez-Morales AJ. Facing Mpox (former Monkeypox) in Latin America: The example of Peru and its vulnerable healthcare system. Vaccines (Basel). 2022;**11**(1):10. DOI: 10.3390/vaccines11010010

[4] Amer F, Khalil HES, Elahmady M, ElBadawy NE, Zahran WA, Abdelnasser M, et al. Mpox: Risks and approaches to prevention. Journal of Infection and Public Health. 2023;**16**(6):901-910

[5] Antinori S, Casalini G, Giacomelli A, Rodriguez-Morales AJ. Update on Mpox: A brief narrative review. Le Infezioni in Medicina. 2023;**31**(3):269-276

[6] Rodriguez-Morales AJ, Schlagenhauf P. Zoonoses and travel medicine: "one world--one health". Travel Medicine and Infectious Disease. 2014;**12**(6 Pt A):555-556

[7] Leon-Figueroa DA, Bonilla-Aldana DK, Pachar M, Romani L, Saldana-Cumpa HM, Anchay-Zuloeta C, et al. The never-ending global emergence of viral zoonoses after COVID-19? The rising concern of monkeypox in Europe, North America and beyond. Travel Medicine and Infectious Disease. 2022;**49**:102362

[8] Parvez MK, Parveen S. Evolution and emergence of pathogenic viruses: Past, present, and future. Intervirology. 2017;**60**(1-2):1-7

[9] Young PR. Arboviruses: A family on the move. Advances in Experimental Medicine and Biology. 2018;**1062**:1-10

[10] Soni S, Gill VJS, Anusheel SJ, Chhabra J, Gill GJS, et al. Dengue, chikungunya, and Zika: The causes and threats of emerging and re-emerging arboviral diseases. Cureus. 2023;**15**(7):e41717

[11] Abdelrahman AHM, Mekhemer GAH, Sidhom PA, El-Tayeb MA, Khan S, Ibrahim MAA. Drug repurposing investigation for combating Ebola virus disease: Database mining, docking calculations, molecular dynamics, and density functional theory study. ChemistryOpen. 2025:e202500348. DOI: 10.1002/open.202500348 [In press]

[12] Bisanzio D, Bosa HK, Bakamutumaho B, Nasimiyu C, Atwine D, Kyabayinze D, et al. Modeling case burden and duration of Sudan Ebola virus disease outbreak in Uganda, 2022. Emerging Infectious Diseases. 2025;**31**(9):1829-1832

[13] Checchi F, Eamer G, Katshitshi J, Robles Dios L, Kai A, Warsame A. Effect of a safe and dignified burial intervention on Ebola virus transmission in the eastern Democratic Republic of the Congo, 2018-19: A propensity score analysis. The Lancet Global Health. 2025;**13**(9):e1617-e1e26

[14] Durante D, Murugesh V, Kalanquin T, Gaisina IN, Rong L, Moore TW. Small molecule drug discovery for Ebola virus disease. RSC. Medicinal Chemistry. 2025. DOI: 10.1039/d5md00533g [In press]

[15] Matson MJ, Chertow DS, Munster VJ. Ebola virus disease: Uniquely challenging among the viral hemorrhagic fevers. Open Forum Infectious Diseases. 2025;**12**(8):ofaf464

[16] Shrivastava SR, Bobhate PS. Extending mental health support to the survivors of Ebola virus disease by overcoming challenges. Germs. 2025;**15**(1):83-87

[17] Umar SK, Diggle MA. The Ebola virus - going beyond the bleeding edge. Journal of Medical Microbiology. 2025;**74**(7):001998. DOI: 10.1099/jmm.0.001998

[18] Wang C, Zhang X, Bai Y, Liu H, Liu X, Cao C. Septin9 promotes viral replication by interacting with Ebola virus VP35 to regulate inclusion body formation. Sheng Wu Gong Cheng Xue Bao. 2025;**41**(8):3228-3240

[19] Zhao J, Zhang B, Vogel O, Walker BW, Ma LW, Wagner ND, et al. The biophysical basis for karyopherin-dependent Ebola virus VP24 nuclear transport. Viruses. 2025;**17**(8):1051. DOI: 10.3390/v17081051

[20] Zhou J, Zhang X, Yao Y, Xie Y, Li F, Wang W, et al. Recombinant live attenuated measles virus-based vaccines inducing comprehensive protection against Ebola and Marburg viruses. Molecular Therapy. 2025. DOI: 10.1016/j.ymthe.2025.08.022 [In press]

[21] Mayer SV, Tesh RB, Vasilakis N. The emergence of arthropod-borne viral diseases: A global prospective on dengue, chikungunya and zika fevers. Acta Tropica. 2017;**166**:155-163

[22] Bittar C, Machado RRG, Comelis MT, Bueno LM, Morielle-Versute E, Beguelini MR, et al. Lack of serological and molecular evidence of arbovirus infections in bats from Brazil. PLoS One. 2018;**13**(11):e0207010

[23] Guth S, Hanley KA, Althouse BM, Boots M. Ecological processes underlying the emergence of novel enzootic cycles: Arboviruses in the neotropics as a case study. PLoS Neglected Tropical Diseases. 2020;**14**(8):e0008338

[24] Farahat RA, Abdelaal A, Umar TP, El-Sakka AA, Benmelouka AY, Albakri K, et al. The emergence of SARS-CoV-2 omicron subvariants: Current situation and future trends. Le Infezioni in Medicina. 2022;**30**(4):480-494

[25] Barbosa AN, Chebabo A, Starling C, Perez C, Cunha CA, de Luna D, et al. Pan-American guidelines for the treatment of SARS-CoV-2/COVID-19: A joint evidence-based guideline of the Brazilian Society of Infectious Diseases (SBI) and the Pan-American Association of Infectious Diseases (API). Annals of Clinical Microbiology and Antimicrobials. 2023;**22**(1):67

[26] Carrion-Nessi FS, Ascanio LC, Pineda-Arape AG, Omana-Avila OD, Mendoza-Millan DL, Romero SR, et al. New daily persistent headache after SARS-CoV-2 infection in Latin America: A cross-sectional study. BMC Infectious Diseases. 2023;**23**(1):877

[27] Rodriguez-Morales AJ, Barbosa AN, Cimerman S. Editorial: New therapeutic approaches for SARS-CoV-2/COVID-19. Frontiers in Immunology. 2023;**14**:1276279

[28] Valderrama-Beltran S, Cuervo-Rojas J, Martinez-Vernaza S,

Alvarez-Moreno CA, Rodriguez-Morales AJ. SARS-CoV-2 vaccination strategies: Should the extended dosing interval strategy be implemented in future pandemics? Travel Medicine and Infectious Disease. 2023;**56**:102650

[29] Aguilar-Martinez SL, Sandoval-Pena GA, Molina-Mora JA, Tsukayama-Cisneros P, Diaz-Velez C, Aguilar-Gamboa FR, et al. Genomic and phylogenetic characterisation of SARS-CoV-2 genomes isolated in patients from Lambayeque region, Peru. Tropical Medicine and Infectious Diseases. 2024;**9**(2):46. DOI: 10.3390/tropicalmed9020046

[30] Nawab M, Riaz SK, Ismail E, Ahamed A, Tariq A, Malik MFA, et al. Integrated approach for detection of SARS-CoV-2 and its variant by utilizing LAMP and ARMS-PCR. Annals of Clinical Microbiology and Antimicrobials. 2024;**23**(1):11

[31] Thomas LF, Rushton J, Bukachi SA, Falzon LC, Howland O, Fèvre EM. Cross-sectoral zoonotic disease surveillance in Western Kenya: Identifying drivers and barriers within a resource constrained setting. Frontiers in Veterinary Science. 2021;**8**:658454

[32] Hsu VP, Haessler S, Banach DB, Batshon LJ, Branch-Elliman W, Dumyati G, et al. SHEA position statement on pandemic preparedness for policymakers: Introduction and overview. Infection Control and Hospital Epidemiology. 2024;**45**(7):801-803

[33] Kufoof L, Hajjeh R, Al Nsour M, Saad R, Bélorgeot V, Abubakar A, et al. Learning from COVID-19: What would it take to Be better prepared in the eastern Mediterranean region? JMIR Public Health and Surveillance. 2024;**10**:e40491

[34] Humos L, Basha H, Saleh W, Awashreh F, Baradiea A, Salhab E, et al. Implementing one health in Palestine: Mapping ministerial mechanisms for pandemic preparedness, zoonotic disease control, and inter-sectoral collaboration. One Health. 2025;**20**:101100

[35] Calouro R, de Sousa T, Saraiva S, Fernandes D, Mourao AV, Igrejas G, et al. Tick-borne pathogens in companion animals and zoonotic risk in Portugal: A one health surveillance approach. Microorganisms. 2025;**13**(8):1774. DOI: 10.3390/microorganisms13081774

[36] deJonge ML, Yuen S, Simard L, Sabiston CM. One-on-one and group-based physical activity intervention compared to a waitlist control for post-secondary student mental health and social well-being: A 3-arm parallel randomized controlled trial protocol. PLoS One. 2025;**20**(8):e0330851

[37] Di Guardo G. Reporting of West Nile virus: A one health concern? The Veterinary Record. 2025;**197**(5):207-208

[38] Elbehiry A, Marzouk E. Staphylococci in livestock: Molecular epidemiology, antimicrobial resistance, and translational strategies for one health protection. Veterinary Sciences. 2025;**12**(8):757. DOI: 10.3390/vetsci12080757

[39] Elton L, Mateos AD, Frosini SM, Jepson R, Rofael S, McHugh TD, et al. A metagenomic approach to one health surveillance of antimicrobial resistance in a UK veterinary Centre. Microbial Genomics. 2025;**11**(9):001471. DOI: 10.1099/mgen.0.001471

[40] Ferrinho R, Ferrinho P. Expanding the public health response to economic warfare through a one health integration. The International Journal of Health Planning and Management. 2025. DOI: 10.1002/hpm.70020 [In press]

[41] Freitas AR, de Franca DA, Kmetiuk LB, Martini R, Delai RR, Pimpao CT, et al. One health approach to *Coxiella burnetii*: First serosurvey of owners and dogs living on oceanic islands and mainland seashore areas of Brazil. Frontiers in Public Health. 2025;**13**:1643457

[42] Howren MB, Hansen JR. The one big beautiful bill act-implications for rural health care. JAMA. 2025;**334**(13):1143-1144. DOI: 10.1001/jama.2025.13518

[43] Ibeagha-Awemu EM, Omonijo FA, Piche LC, Vincent AT. Alternatives to antibiotics for sustainable livestock production in the context of the one health approach: Tackling a common foe. Frontiers in Veterinary Science. 2025;**12**:1605215

[44] Jibowu MH, Chung R, Tang NL, Guo S, Lawton LA, Sullivan BJ, et al. Leishmania in Texas: A contemporary one health scoping review of vectors, reservoirs, and human health. Biology (Basel). 2025;**14**(8):999. DOI: 10.3390/biology14080999

[45] Kavulavu BM, Omwenga EO, Nyangiri OA, Nyerere AK, Too RJ, Matey EJ, et al. One health approach unravels worrying antimicrobial resistance patterns: A cross-sectional study in Kisii, Kenya. PLoS One. 2025;**20**(9):e0331389

[46] Mena-Vasquez J, Marco-Fuertes A, Culhane M, Torremorell M. Emerging threats of HPAI H5N1 clade 2.3.4.4b in swine: Knowledge gaps and the imperative for a one health approach. Frontiers in Veterinary Science. 2025;**12**:1648878

[47] Mihu ML, Novac CS, Craciun S, Fit NI, Bouari CM, Nadas GC, et al. Urinary multidrug-resistant Klebsiella pneumoniae: Essential oil countermeasures in a one health case report. Microorganisms. 2025;**13**(8):1807. DOI: 10.3390/microorganisms13081807

[48] Ortiz-Millan G. One health in a globalized world: Challenges and responses to zoonotic threats. Global Bioethics. 2025;**36**(1):2550805

[49] Taylor L. One billion people have mental health conditions, WHO says. BMJ. 2025;**390**:r1860

[50] Awaidy SA, Al HH. Zoonotic diseases in Oman: Successes, challenges, and future directions. Vector Borne and Zoonotic Diseases. 2020;**20**(1):1-9

[51] Gallego-Pérez DF, Declercq E, Saper RB, Barnes LL, Wardle J. Characterizing therapeutic pluralism policies in Latin America: A qualitative content analysis. Journal of Complementary and Integrative Medicine. 2023;**29**(6-7):439-450

[52] Zinsstag J, Utzinger J, Probst-Hensch N, Shan L, Zhou XN. Towards integrated surveillance-response systems for the prevention of future pandemics. Infectious Diseases of Poverty. 2020;**9**(1):140

[53] Gamble A, Olarte-Castillo XA, Whittaker GR. Backyard zoonoses: The roles of companion animals and peri-domestic wildlife. Science Translational Medicine. 2023;**15**(718):eadj0037

[54] Schmiedel S, Wolf T. Viral hemorrhagic fever (VHF) with a potential for human-to-human transmission. Deutsche Medizinische Wochenschrift. 2025;**150**(13):758-771

[55] Yao W, Yang Z, Lou X, Mao H, Yan H, Zhang Y. Simultaneous detection of Ebola virus and pathogens associated with hemorrhagic fever by an oligonucleotide microarray. Frontiers in Microbiology. 2021;**12**:713372

[56] Boshevska G, Emmerich P, von Possel R, Jancheska E, Buzharova T, Kochinski D, et al. Genomic characterization of Orthonairovirus haemorrhagiae (Crimean-Congo hemorrhagic fever virus) outbreak in North Macedonia. Microbiology Resource Announcements. 2024;**13**(12):e0074924

[57] O'Hearn AE, Voorhees MA, Fetterer DP, Wauquier N, Coomber MR, Bangura J, et al. Serosurveillance of viral pathogens circulating in West Africa. Virology Journal. 2016;**13**(1):163

[58] Mariano MC, Hvasta MG, Dowd KA, Huang WC, Jung HS, Evanson LR, et al. Design of Hyperglycosylated Zika Virus E Proteins that focus antibody recognition on the complex E dimer epitope. ACS Chemical Biology. 2025;**20**(9):2105-2119. DOI: 10.1021/acschembio.5c00253

[59] Harding AT, Zhang Y, Chen JJ, Antonucci JM, Richards A, Leger V et al. Oxidative Stress and Interferon Signaling Drive Differential Pathogenesis of Ancestral and Contemporary Zika Viruses in Human Cerebral Organoids. bioRxiv; 2025

[60] Lebov JF, Nason M, Stolka KB, Ximenes R, Mussi-Pinhata MM, Moye J, et al. Zika in infants and pregnancy (ZIP) study: Results from a prospective international cohort study of prenatal Zika virus infection and adverse fetal and infant outcomes. BMC Pregnancy and Childbirth. 2025;**25**(1):903

[61] Zhang S, Wu J, Wang D, Song J, Li Y, Yin C, et al. The first imported case of Zika virus infection - Shandong Province, China, 2025. China CDC Weekly. 2025;**7**(30):1004-1008

[62] Kleber Rodrigues Lima W, Zeneida Gomes Parente Alves Lima C, Kleber Gomes Parente Alves Lima V, Reis Rosario W, Goncalves Lima-Neto L, Dos Santos Correia MT, et al. Druggable targets in Zika virus: A systematic review of therapeutic opportunities in Brazil. Current Topics in Medicinal Chemistry. 2025. DOI: 10.2174/0115680266388856250811094000 [In press]

[63] Yan Y, Wang J, Yang H, Yang Y, Yuan L, Tang C, et al. The modified mRNA vaccine protects immunocompromised AG129 mice from lethal challenge and multi-tissue infection by Zika virus. Emerg. Microbes and Infection. 2025;**14**(1):2556729

[64] Kikuta K, Hernandez CJ, de Abranches AD, Damasceno L, de Britto JA, Duarte CJ, et al. Academic and social-behavioral assessment in a prospective cohort of normocephalic school-aged children with antenatal Zika virus exposure. International Journal of Infectious Diseases. 2025:108026. DOI: 10.1016/j.ijid.2025.108026

[65] Seo SH, Choi JA, Yang E, Park H, Jung DI, Kim JO, et al. Mouse strain-dependent neutralizing antibody responses to Zika virus vaccines. Journal of Microbiology. 2025;**63**(8):e2504005

[66] Westphal C, Stanhope S, Cooper W, Wang C. A mathematical model for Zika virus disease: Intervention methods and control of affected pregnancies. Mathematical Biosciences and Engineering. 2025;**22**(8):1956-1979

[67] Lourenco MR, Christoff RR, Rabello T, Paura LG, Ferreira J, Mendes FA, et al. Postnatal Zika virus infection increases seizure susceptibility and disrupts cortical organization and GABAergic interneuron positioning in mice. Neuroscience. 2025;**585**:125-132. DOI: 10.1016/j.neuroscience.2025.08.026

[68] Acharya SS, Rout PR, Barad LM, Dansana J, Gadtya A, Meher BR, et al.

Visible light-driven photocatalyst-free cascade synthesis of functionalized benzopyrans as inhibitors of chikungunya nsPs and Zika NS2B-NS3. Organic & Biomolecular Chemistry. 2025;**23**(37):8465-8473. DOI: 10.1039/d5ob01283j

[69] Loisel L, Raquin V, Ratinier M, Ezanno P, Beaunee G. Intra-vector infection dynamics challenge how to model the extrinsic incubation period for major arboviruses: Dengue, Zika, and chikungunya. PLoS Computational Biology. 2025;**21**(8):e1013393

[70] Salazar Florez JE, Restrepo BN, Freitas LP, Carabali M, Jaramillo Ramirez GI, Balaguera CG, et al. Spatio-temporal analysis of the distribution and co-circulation of dengue, chikungunya, and Zika in Medellin, Colombia, from 2013 to 2021. PLoS Neglected Tropical Diseases. 2025;**19**(9):e0013470

[71] Willcox AC, Gobillot TA, Kikawa C, Baumgarten NE, Stoddard CI, Sung K, et al. Identification of AMOTL2 as an antiviral factor that enhances the human type I interferon response against Zika virus. Proceedings of the National Academy of Sciences of the United States of America. 2025;**122**(36):e2507955122

[72] Abramov DM, Silva DSE, Rios AS, Hedin-Pereira C, Costa A, Moreira MEL. The role of neurophysiology in investigating neuropathology of vertical Zika virus infection. Reviews in Medical Virology. 2025;**35**(5):e70068

[73] Rifakis PM, Benitez JA, De-la-Paz-Pineda J, Rodriguez-Morales AJ. Epizootics of yellow fever in Venezuela (2004-2005): An emerging zoonotic disease. Annals of the New York Academy of Sciences. 2006;**1081**:57-60

[74] Ortiz-Martinez Y, Patino-Barbosa AM, Rodriguez-Morales AJ. Yellow fever in the Americas: The growing concern about new epidemics. F1000Res. 2017;**6**:398

[75] Srivastava S, Dhoundiyal S, Kumar S, Kaur A, Khatib MN, Gaidhane S, et al. Yellow fever: Global impact, epidemiology, pathogenesis, and integrated prevention approaches. Le Infezioni in Medicina. 2024;**32**(4):434-450

[76] Alvarez-Moreno CA, Rodriguez-Morales AJ. Challenges of the current yellow fever outbreak in Colombia. Lancet. 2025;**405**(10497):2273

[77] Reno E, Quan NG, Franco-Paredes C, Chastain DB, Chauhan L, Rodriguez-Morales AJ, et al. Prevention of yellow fever in travellers: An update. The Lancet Infectious Diseases. 2020;**20**(6):e129-ee37

[78] Forero-Delgadillo AJ, Morales-Olivera JA, Celis-Guzman JF, Zapata-Diaz OE, Gonzalez-Varona GA, Acevedo-Bedoya CA, et al. Colombian consensus on the care of critically ill patients with suspected or confirmed severe yellow fever. The Lancet Regional Health. 2025;**48**:101144

[79] Angerami RN, Socorro Souza Chaves TD, Rodriguez-Morales AJ. Yellow fever outbreaks in South America: Current epidemiology, legacies of the recent past and perspectives for the near future. New Microbes New Infections. 2025;**65**:101580

[80] Sanchez-Rojas IC, Solarte-Jimenez CL, Chamorro-Velazco EC, Diaz-Llerena GE, Arevalo CD, Cuasquer-Posos OL, et al. Yellow fever in Putumayo, Colombia, 2024. New Microbes New Infections. 2025;**64**:101572

[81] Rodriguez-Morales AJ, Sah R, Silva-Ramos CR, Pava-Garzon DM. Challenges

in emerging and reemerging Arboviral diseases: The examples of Oropouche and yellow fever. Pathogens. 2025;**14**(7)

[82] Chaves T, Orduna T, Lepetic A, Macchi A, Verbanaz S, Risquez A, et al. Yellow fever in Brazil: Epidemiological aspects and implications for travelers. Travel Medicine and Infectious Disease. 2018;**23**:1-3

[83] Rodriguez-Morales AJ, Alhazmi AH, Katime A, Hameed AA, Morales A, Lepetic AC, et al. Yellow fever in South America - a plea for action and call for prevention also in travelers from SLAMVI, ESGITM, EVASG, ALEIMC, GEPI-SEIMC, SEMEVI, and CMTZMV-ACIN. Travel Medicine and Infectious Disease. 2025;**67**:102871

[84] Rodriguez-Morales AJ, Bonilla-Aldana DK, Suarez JA, Franco-Paredes C, Forero-Pena DA, Mattar S, et al. Yellow fever reemergence in Venezuela - implications for international travelers and Latin American countries during the COVID-19 pandemic. Travel Medicine and Infectious Disease. 2021;**44**:102192

[85] Antonucci J, Gehrke L. Cerebral organoid models for neurotropic viruses. ACS Infectious Diseases. 2019;**5**(12):1976-1979

[86] Al-Obaidi MMJ, Bahadoran A, Wang SM, Manikam R, Raju CS, Sekaran SD. Disruption of the blood brain barrier is vital property of neurotropic viral infection of the central nervous system. Acta Virologica. 2018;**62**(1):16-27

[87] Abdullahi AM, Sarmast ST, Singh R. Molecular biology and epidemiology of neurotropic viruses. Cureus. 2020;**12**(8):e9674

[88] Sievers BL, Siegers JY, Cadènes JM, Hyder S, Sparaciari FE, Claes F, et al. Smart markets: Harnessing the potential of new technologies for endemic and emerging infectious disease surveillance in traditional food markets. Journal of Virology. 2024;**98**(2):e0168323

[89] Asante J, Noreddin A, El Zowalaty ME. Systematic review of important bacterial zoonoses in Africa in the last decade in light of the 'one health' concept. Pathogens. 2019;**8**(2)

[90] Hassan OA, de Balogh K, Winkler AS. One health early warning and response system for zoonotic diseases outbreaks: Emphasis on the involvement of grassroots actors. Veterinary Medicine and Science. 2023;**9**(4):1881-1889

[91] Whitehead J, Olliaro P, Lang T, Horby P. Trial design for evaluating novel treatments during an outbreak of an infectious disease. Clinical Trials. 2016;**13**(1):31-38

[92] Qiu Y, Guitian J, Webster JP, Musallam I, Haider N, Drewe JA, et al. Global prioritization of endemic zoonotic diseases for conducting surveillance in domestic animals to protect public health. Philosophical Transactions of the Royal Society of London. Series B, Biological Sciences. 1887;**2023**(378):20220407

[93] Richardson T, Johnston AM, Draper H. A systematic review of Ebola treatment trials to assess the extent to which they adhere to ethical guidelines. PLoS One. 2017;**12**(1):e0168975

[94] Naeem I, Siddiqi S, Siddiqui AR, Hasan R. Exploring stakeholders' experiences and perceptions regarding barriers to effective surveillance of communicable diseases in a rural district of Pakistan: A qualitative study. BMJ Open. 2022;**12**(11):e067031

[95] Kabajaasi O, Schilling S, Akugizibwe M, Horby PW, Hart P, Sigfrid L, et al. Involve those who are managing these outbreaks': Stakeholders' perspectives on the barriers and facilitators to the implementation of clinical management guidelines for high-consequence infectious diseases in Uganda-a thematic network analysis. BMJ Public Health. 2025;**3**(1):e001165

[96] Ahmed MM, Oweidat M, Okesanya OJ, Alaswad M, Abdelbar SMM, Gill P, et al. Barriers to pediatric emergency care in low-resource settings: A narrative review. Sage Open Pediatrics. 2025;**12**:30502225251336861

Chapter 2

Perspective Chapter: One Health Approach to Zoonotic Disease Control – Collaboration and Integration across Sectors

Monalisa Mohanty, Sutapa Rath, Gayatree Nayak, Preetam Kumar Kar and Jeebanjyoti Mishra

Abstract

Zoonotic diseases account for 60% of reported infectious cases of animal origin, posing a major global health threat. Outbreaks such as Ebola, severe acute respiratory syndrome (SARS), Middle East respiratory syndrome (MERS), Nipah, Zika, and COVID-19 highlight the urgent need for an integrated disease prevention strategy. The One Health approach, endorsed by the World Health Organization (WHO), the Food and Agriculture Organization of the United Nations (FAO), and the World Organization for Animal Health (WOAH), bridges human, animal, and environmental health sectors to mitigate transmission risks through cross-sectoral collaboration. This chapter examines the One Health framework's evolution, principles, and implementation challenges. It evaluates successful case studies from Thailand and the United States and identifies major barriers such as governance fragmentation, inadequate funding, and limited data sharing. Despite challenges, One Health has demonstrated effectiveness in disease prevention through enhanced surveillance, interdisciplinary collaboration, and equitable healthcare access. Case studies highlight the impact of coordinated monitoring, joint research, and veterinary public health initiatives in mitigating zoonotic threats. The One Health framework offers a sustainable, long-term solution for zoonotic disease control, requiring political commitment, intersectoral coordination, and community engagement. Strengthening global policies, securing funding, and fostering interdisciplinary partnerships will accelerate innovation, enhance disease resilience, and safeguard public health.

Keywords: one health, zoonotic diseases, multisectoral collaboration, surveillance systems, global health security, interdisciplinary approach

1. Introduction

About 60% of globally reported emerging infections originate from the animal world. In the last three decades, over 30 new human pathogens have been detected, three-quarters of which originated in domestic and wild animals. Human activities like agriculture, animal trade, livestock farming, urbanization, encroachment into wild areas, extractive industries, and ongoing climate change further complicate the entwined human, animal, and environmental health.

The One Health concept, introduced at the beginning of the 2000s, explores these close links between human, animal, and environmental health that demand cul-de-sac collaboration, communication, as well as coordination between the relevant sectors. One Health is "an integrated, unifying approach to balance and optimize the health of people, animals, and ecosystems" [1]. According to the definition given by the One Health Initiative Task Force, One Health is "the collaborative efforts of multiple disciplines working locally, nationally, and globally, to attain optimal health for people, animals, and our environment", signifying human health cannot be separated from animal health [2].

In the last few decades, humanity has encountered recurring waves of emerging as well as reemerging infectious diseases, often lacking treacherous counterdefences. Western Africa faced the Ebola outbreak between 2013 and 2016, causing an excess of 11,000 deaths; many viral hemorrhagic fevers with high morbidity and mortality rates; the severe acute respiratory syndrome coronavirus (SARS-CoV) outbreak in 2003, and the middle east respiratory syndrome coronavirus (MERS-CoV) in 2012, have led to uncountable deaths. In addition, the Nipah virus and Zika virus, causative agents of lethal encephalitis and neonatal malformation, have also led to global public health emergencies [3]. The COVID-19 pandemic is another harbinger that warns of the need to reconsider and reevaluate the current health care archetypes expeditiously. Human health can no longer be an isolated entity; rather, it should be contemplated as a part of the animal, plant, and environmental biosphere.

A blueprint list of priority diseases has been launched by the World Health Organization (WHO) to expedite research and development (R&D) for these pathogens. The latest blueprint issued by the WHO in February 2018, unveiled the most priority diseases, which included Ebola virus disease (EVD), Lassa fever virus (LF), Marburg virus disease (MVD), Crimean Congo hemorrhagic fever (CCHF), Middle East respiratory syndrome (MERS) and severe acute respiratory syndrome (SARS), Nipah and henipaviral diseases, Rift Valley fever (RVF), Zika, and "Disease X", a yet unknown disease [4]. One Health has six focus areas that include laboratory services, neglected tropical diseases, antimicrobial resistance, control of zoonotic diseases, food safety, and environmental health [4]. This approach, therefore mobilizes multiple sectors as well as communities simultaneously at different tiers of the society to work together and foster well-being as well as handle threats against health and ecosystem, while addressing important issues like collective need for clean water, safe and nutritious food, energy and air, tackling on climate change, and promoting sustainable development.

1.1 History: The evolution of "One Health: Concept to Concrete"

The concept of One Health can be traced back ages to the ancient Greek philosopher Aristotle, who emphasized the interdependence of human health on the ecosystem; these principles have been practiced from time immortal [5, 6]. In the nineteenth century, Rudolf Virchow notedly remarked, "Between animal and human medicine there is no dividing line-nor should there be" [7].

In the mid-twentieth century, a veterinary surgeon in the United States, Calvin Schwabe, suggested the concept of "One Medicine". He highlighted the integrated, cross-disciplinary perspective with involvement of social sciences and better communication skills to improve working together with the community in efforts to control infectious diseases [8].

The SARS-CoV-1 emergence in the early 2000s prompted the Wildlife Conservation Society (WCS) to formulate the 'Manhattan Principles of Conservation' in 2004, serving as the foundation for the twenty-first-century One Health movement. These principles particularly called for an integrated view of interactions among humans and animals and recognized the unpredictable nature of emerging microbes as well as the demand for transnational cooperation and efforts in response to prevent or mitigate epidemics and pandemics [9]. The WCS introduced the term "One World-One Health" at the conference to entwine both medicine and ecosystem health, and listed 12 principles to establish a better holistic approach to prevent epidemics and establish the integrity of the ecosystem to benefit people, domesticated animals, and biodiversity [10].

The One Health Tripartite collaboration, established in 2010, of the World Organization for Animal Health (WOAH), the Food and Agriculture Organization of the United Nations (FAO), and the WHO had taken multiple steps to in human-animal-environment biosphere for global health security and provided a structured approach against zoonoses, antimicrobial resistance, and food safety [11]. Over time, with further evolution of the concept, the latest being "One Health Joint Plan of Action" for 2022 till 2026 by the Quadripartite, a consortium consisting of WHO, the Food and Agriculture Organization of the United Nations (FAO), the World Organization for Animal Health (WOAH), and the United Nations Environment Program (UNEP) which are the principal multilateral agencies focused on human, animal and environmental health [12].

1.2 One health: Core principles and frame board

Key principles of one-health include:

1. Equity among various sectors and disciplines;

2. Sociopolitical and multicultural parity (the doctrine that all people are equal and deserve equal rights and opportunities) and inclusion and engagement of communities and marginalized voices;

3. Socioecological equilibrium seeking a harmonious balance within human-animal-environment interaction as well as acknowledging the significance of biodiversity, accessing sufficient natural space and resources, and the internal value of all living things in the ecosystem;

4. Stewardship and human responsibility for change of behavior and adoption of sustainable solutions to value animal welfare and complete integrity of the ecosystem, hence securing the well-being of the current as well as upcoming generation; and

5. Transdisciplinary and multisectoral collaboration, including relevant disciplines, with both modern and traditional forms of knowledge and a broad array of perspectives [1].

A pictorial depiction of the One Health concept is given below in **Figure 1**.

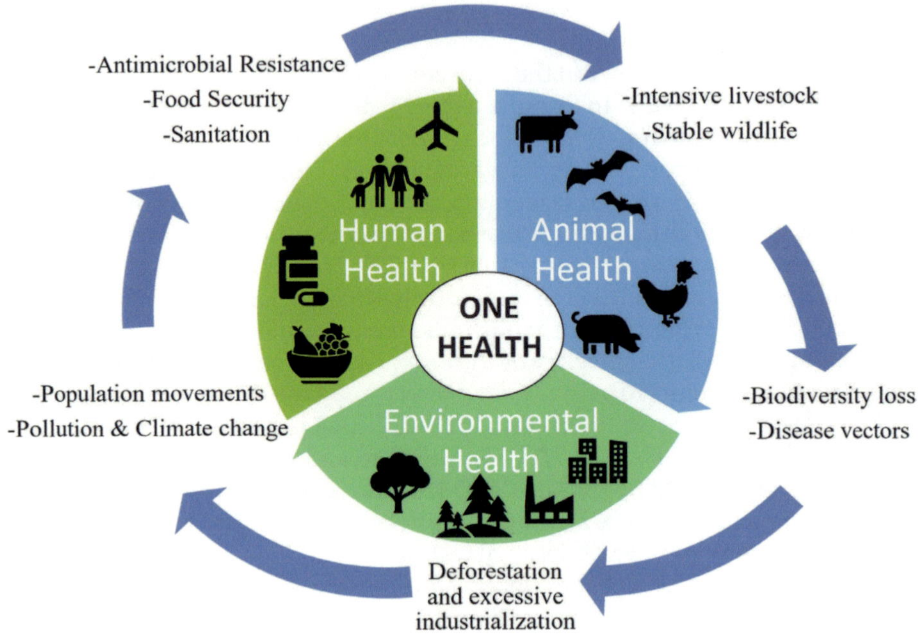

Figure 1.
The One Health Paradigm: Connecting Human, Animal, and Environmental Well-Being.

1.3 Role of various stakeholders and multisectoral collaboration

The One Health approach depends on multisectoral collaboration involving various stakeholders working in harmony with each other.

1. *Multilateral Organizations*

The international bodies, WHO, OIE, UNEP, and FAO, form the quadripartite with the greatest responsibilities of global health, and have recognized that for health security protection and promotion of overall global well-being, disciplinary and jurisdictional boundaries need to be foregone and governance structures need to be established to solve current intricate health challenges.

2. *Regional networks and international donors*

In conjunction with the above international bodies, multisectoral regional systems are emerging, which enable improved disease surveillance along with joint approaches for aligned interventions across country borders. The East African Integrated Disease Surveillance Network, for example, pursues the motto of reducing morbidity and mortality due to frequent communicable diseases in Uganda, Tanzania, and Kenya. Another organization, the Southern African Centre for Infectious Disease Surveillance, which is a One Health center, on a virtual mode, linking academic as well as research institutions in South Africa for infectious disease surveillance. The Mekong Basin Disease Surveillance network is one such paradigm of old cross-border collaborative relations involving China, Cambodia, Myanmar, the Lao People's Democratic Republic, Vietnam and Thailand that tries to control outbreaks of disease through reporting, collaborative regional surveillance, joint outbreak detections as well as capacity building, with inceptive support from the Rockefeller Foundation. Likewise, the Middle East Consortium of Infectious Disease Surveillance, which was started in 2001, works at multiple levels, starting from a smaller community to the larger region, working toward the detection as well as control of infectious diseases. The CORDS network (Connecting Organizations for Regional Disease Surveillance) started in 2013, joins together all such existing regional networks of the world, and promotes global exchanges of best practices, tools, strategies, training courses, innovations, case studies, and technical data to improve disease surveillance worldwide.

3. *Ministries, policymakers, and collaborating organizations*

Ministries, together with policymakers, must secure health care systems that are functioning, and allow for adequate building capacity, resource utilization, and competence at national levels, along with formulation of appropriate, robust acts, policies, and regulations as well as guidelines on disease surveillance, control, and prevention. The key ministries that can ensure implementation of One Health services can be health, agriculture, and environment ministries along with the ministries of finance, home affairs, education, and the Prime Minister's office, which often oversee government authorities are key stake holders and the disaster management department can also play an important role during outbreaks.

4. *Universities*

Universities can pitch in to enhance all stages of the One Health process, encouraging and stimulating field research, and serve as cardinal catalysts of One Health collaborations in multiple sectors like environmental sciences, wildlife, and agriculture. They can exemplify the note worthiness of this research, help in prioritizing and in assembling appropriate stakeholders that can further help translate knowledge into action, and provide priming and expertise in one-health problem solving, and come up with unbiased expert opinion. In 2007, the Canadian Cooperative Wildlife Health Centre (CCWHC), an academic organization that coordinates the country's national wildlife health surveillance program and comprises all of the nation's veterinary colleges, utilized the knowledge of wildlife health and disease to improve human health and the health of domestic animals. It also provides information and educational programs to the general public and consultation to both the government and non-government organizations.

5. *Non-governmental organizations*

Non-governmental organizations (NGOs) are involved in:

- the generation, management, and utilization of knowledge
- resource mobilization
- capacity building
- hands-on execution.

They play a major role in advocating and promoting pertinent global health issues and problems. In collaboration with other contributors, these bodies convey and put forward One Health ideas of critical importance, which can include:

- zoonoses
- disease and conflict mitigation in wildlife
- local and global food security
- human– domestic animal interface
- policies
- commodity trade.

NGOs particularly foster partnerships among various tiers of the system that include governments, general communities, universities, and development agencies. One such instance includes the PREDICT project, which includes the segment of the United States Agency for International Development (USAID) Emerging Pandemic Threats program. The PREDICT project, under the USAID, develops predictive modeling approaches for the identification of hotspot regions where experts from different specialties like epidemiology, virology, genetics, informatics, and veterinary medicine work in active collaboration in hotspots in 20 developing countries, focusing on surveillance and improving diagnostic capacities at human-animal interfaces at areas of common cross-species transmission [13].

6. *Communities*

Communities, especially ones with rural and indigenous people in nature's vicinity, form the essence of One Health. Healthy wildlife, humans, and the domesticated animals on whom people depend for their sustenance can help mitigate crucial public health threats while facilitating environmental management. Hence, community involvement and empowerment are pivotal for the triumph of One Health initiatives [14].

2. Multisectoral collaboration

Multisectoral collaboration is key to the One Health approach, which aims to reduce zoonotic diseases by promoting combined efforts between human, animal, and environmental health sectors. This collaboration involves partnerships among veterinarians, medical professionals, ecologists, policymakers, and researchers to identify and address the interconnected factors contributing to zoonotic transmission [15–17].

Various collaboration mechanisms may include collaborative research involving professionals from human health, veterinary health, and environmental sciences to investigate zoonotic pathogens and their transmission dynamics, integrating surveillance data from human health systems, veterinary monitoring, and environmental assessments to identify and respond to emerging public health threats and developing unified policies that address zoonotic disease risks across sectors, ensuring coordinated action. The human health sector may contribute through robust public health monitoring systems for early detection of zoonotic outbreaks, education, awareness among the community about preventive measures, and advancements in the management of zoonotic diseases through research and development. The animal health sector may contribute through the surveillance and control of diseases among livestock and wildlife to prevent cross-species transmission, as well as implementing multiple practices to reduce the risk of zoonotic disease spread in agricultural and wildlife settings. The environmental health sector may contribute by identifying ecological factors that give rise to the emergence of zoonotic disease, for example, climate change, and promoting sustainable practices like biodiversity conservation to alleviate zoonotic disease risks [1, 15, 17].

2.1 Challenges and barriers in implementing the one health policies

Implementing One Health policies to control and prevent zoonotic diseases in any geographical area faces numerous hurdles and challenges. These result from the breaches in the interdisciplinary collaboration across different sectors like human health, animal husbandry, the agricultural field, and environmental protection. A few of these important key obstacles are discussed below.

1. Fragmented Governance and Policy Incoherence: Fragmented Governance structures and the absence of cohesive policies hinder the effective implementation of One Health policies. In many areas, especially developing countries, there is a marked deficiency of political commitment and robust governance structures to support One Health initiatives. Additionally, disparities in legal frameworks and a lack of harmony among the different regulatory bodies obstructs integrated action against zoonotic diseases [18].

2. Constraints on resources: (i) financial limitations: Substantial funding is essential to execute comprehensive One Health strategies, which is often lacking, particularly in low- and middle-income countries; (ii) shortage of manpower: To date, there is a deficit of both trained professionals in different fields needed for the smooth functioning of One Health approach such as expertise in veterinary public health, environmental science, and epidemiology, and regular training programs, resulting in incoherence to different strategies of One Health [19].

3. Inadequate Surveillance and Data Sharing: Robust surveillance systems are crucial for early detection and prompt response to zoonotic diseases. However, many countries lack integrated surveillance systems across various sectors and are reluctant to share data owing to the privacy concerns of different institutions and political sensitivities, which compromise the efforts of zoonotic disease monitoring [20].

4. Knowledge Gaps and Research Needs: There is a critical need for large-scale studies across the globe that connect human, animal, and environmental health sciences to apprise One Health strategies, but the quandary is that the environmental health considerations are frequently overlooked in zoonotic disease prevention efforts. This might be a major reason for the zoonotic disease outbreaks [21].

5. Low public awareness and engagement: So far, public understanding of the One Health concept and the risks associated with zoonotic diseases remains limited in many parts of the world. Several communities still follow many traditional customs involving animals, which may conflict with various disease control measures, necessitating culturally sensitive engagement strategies. These communities are unaware of the One Health concept or the significance of zoonotic risks, leading to low community engagement for related policies [21].

6. Environmental and Ecological Challenges: Different environmental factors, such as deforestation, climate change, and urbanization, play a pivotal role in the emergence and spillover of zoonotic diseases. However, environmental health is often marginalized in One Health policies, creating a gap in addressing the ecological determinants of disease [20].

7. Political and Economic Pressures: Change in leadership, political priorities, and economic interests can adversely affect the long-term strategies of One Health policies. Industries like agriculture and wildlife trade may resist regulations perceived as economically detrimental, which in turn negatively affect the implementation of these policies [19].

2.2 Zoonotic disease surveillance and monitoring

Zoonotic diseases have emerged as major public health challenges over the years and are responsible for significant economic burdens around the world. It is estimated that the number of new zoonotic cases across the world is about one billion, with 75% ascribing to the emerging infectious diseases and 60% to the bioterror agents causing Middle East respiratory syndrome, Ebola, and avian influenza. According to the World Bank's evaluation, only six zoonotic pandemics were responsible for more than $80 billion in economic losses between 1997 and 1999. The bilateral impact of such infections on humans and animals leads to the vicious cycle of poverty-health deterioration, especially in resource-limited countries. Past experiences from the various zoonotic outbreaks illustrate that effective active surveillance and monitoring systems are the keys to early diagnosis and proactive response to zoonotic diseases. In 2010, the World Health Organization (WHO), the World Organization for Animal Health (WOAH), and the Food and Agriculture Organization (FAO) acknowledged that global multilevel cooperation is essential to curb the threats posed by zoonoses to humans, animals, and the environment [19, 22].

2.2.1 Key components of zoonotic disease surveillance

An integrated multilevel approach is the cornerstone of zoonotic disease surveillance, which includes the following components: (1) Early Detection Systems: To identify any possible outbreaks in animals before they spread to humans. (2) Integrated One Health Approach: Collaboration between human, animal, and environmental health sectors. (3) Data Collection and Reporting System: Real-time reporting of any zoonotic cases using digital tools that help in rapid response to cease the spread of the diseases by taking appropriate measures. (4) Laboratory Networks: Labs with advanced diagnostic platforms to confirm the cases and to track the genetic mutations. (5) Community Engagement: Regular training and learning sessions for at-risk populations such as farmers, butchers, and pet owners [23–25].

2.2.2 Country-wise examples of zoonotic disease outbreaks and control

Many countries have successfully tackled various zoonotic diseases through a well-equipped and dedicated multisectoral integrated approach, setting examples in the world forum. Some of the significant country-wise surveillance systems and One Health operating systems are discussed below.

2.2.2.1 The Thai one health surveillance system

Thailand has been a global leader in One Health, and the Thai One Health Surveillance System is a collaborative approach that integrates human, animal, and environmental health sectors to detect, monitor, and play a crucial role in preventing zoonotic diseases. It involves multiple government agencies, research institutions, and international partners working together to prevent disease outbreaks at the human-animal-environment interface. Thailand has been recognized for its strong One Health framework, which has helped control major zoonotic threats like avian influenza (H5N1), rabies, Nipah virus, and leptospirosis [26, 27].

Key Components of Thailand's One Health Surveillance System:

1. *Multisectoral Collaboration*: Under the aegis of One Health approach, the different sectors work in collaboration, namely:

    a. *Department of Disease Control (DDC)*: Oversees human disease surveillance

    b. *Department of Livestock Development (DLD)*: Monitors animal health and outbreaks

    c. *Department of National Parks Wildlife and Plant Conservation (DNP)*: Monitors environmental and animal health;

    d. *Ministry of Public Health (MoPH)*: Leads public health response and coordination;

    e. *National Institute of Health (NIH), National Institute of Animal Health (NIAH)*: Conducts disease diagnostics and research;

    f. *Academic Institutions and International Organizations*: Collaborate on research and policy (e.g., FAO, WHO, and OIE).

2. *Zoonotic Disease Monitoring and Early Warning Systems:* It helps in the real-time surveillance of high-risk zoonotic diseases. The various examples are - *Event-Based Surveillance (EBS) of Thailand*, where people of all sectors like farmers, veterinarians, and public health workers participate and report on a real-time basis about any unusual animal deaths or human symptoms via mobile apps and community alert systems. Such a system assists the policy makers to be more vigilant, and act promptly to contain and prevent the spread of different zoonotic diseases, such as:

    a. *Avian Influenza (H5N1 and H7N9)*: Continuous poultry and wild bird monitoring

b. *Rabies*: Mass dog vaccinations and bite case reporting

c. *Nipah Virus*: Monitoring fruit bats and pig farms

d. *Leptospirosis*: Surveillance in livestock and flood-prone areas

e. *Brucellosis and Tuberculosis*: Testing dairy cattle and livestock workers

3. Integrated data collection and real-time reporting: Thailand has national disease databases such as

a. *National Epidemiology Surveillance System (NESS)*: Tracks human cases.

b. *National Animal Disease Surveillance System (NADSS)*: Records animal outbreaks.

c. *Thai Rabies Net*: Monitors rabies in real time.

d. *Assistance of AI Surveillance*: Uses AI and big data for outbreak forecasting, which works in an integrated manner for the early prediction of any outbreak.

Examples:

In 2018, cross-sectional data sharing helped in the early detection of an outbreak of H5N1 avian influenza, followed by prompt slaughtering of infected birds and quarantine measures to prevent human infections.

4. *Community engagement and public awareness:* Active involvement of farmers, veterinarians, and the public in zoonotic disease surveillance by implementation of regular training programs for health care providers on zoonotic disease detection, conducting workshops for farmers on biosecurity measures and organizing public awareness campaigns on food safety, rabies prevention, mass dog vaccinations to eliminate rabies death by 2030. As a result, there has been a significant reduction in rabies cases in Thailand in recent years

a. *Emergency Response and Outbreak Control*: Thailand has rapid response teams like

b. *Field Epidemiology Training Program (FETP)*: Trains outbreak response specialists.

c. *Joint animal-human response drills*: prepare for zoonotic pandemics.

d. *Stockpiles of vaccines and antiviral drugs*: enable fast interventions that coordinate with hospitals, veterinary clinics, and research labs to contain outbreaks.

Example:

During the COVID-19 pandemic, Thailand's One Health teams helped to track down and contain outbreaks linked to wildlife trade and live animal markets, preventing further zoonotic spillover.

2.2.2.2 Key components of one health surveillance for zoonotic diseases in the United States

In the United States, this unified approach plays a crucial role in surveillance, prevention, and quick response to zoonotic diseases [28, 29].

1. *Coordinated Surveillance Systems:*

    a. *The Centres for Disease Control and Prevention (CDC), Food and Drug Administration (FDA), and the US Department of Agriculture (USDA)* collaborate to monitor zoonotic disease.

    b. *The National Notifiable Diseases Surveillance System (NNDSS)* tracks human cases of zoonotic diseases.

    c. *The National Animal Health Surveillance System (NAHSS)* monitors diseases in livestock and wildlife, such as COVID-19, and animal surveillance by tracking SARS-CoV-2 infections in animals like mink and deer.

2. *Multiagency Collaborations:*

    a. *National One Health Framework:* The CDC, USDA, and Department of the Interior (DOI) are the leading organizations that execute coordinated efforts.

    b. *National List of Reportable Animal Diseases (NLRAD)*: Ensures timely reporting of animal diseases and Zoonotic Disease Collaboration with State Health Departments: These are the State-level agencies that integrate the data of human and veterinary health.

3. *Wildlife and Livestock Monitoring*: Various organizations, like

    a. *The National Wildlife Health Centre (NWHC)* tracks emerging zoonotic threats in wildlife populations.

    b. *The USDA's Animal and Plant Health Inspection Service (APHIS)* conducts surveillance programs for zoonotic diseases like avian influenza and bovine tuberculosis, helps early detection of any unusual symptoms in animals, and prevents the spillover.

4. *Antimicrobial resistance (AMR) monitoring*: The National Antimicrobial Resistance Monitoring System (NARMS) helps track antibiotic-resistant bacteria in humans, retail meats, and food animals and reduces antibiotic misuse

5. Emerging disease preparedness and response organizations

    a. *One Health Zoonotic Disease Prioritization (OHZDP)* Process: Identifies high-risk zoonotic diseases (e.g., rabies, Lyme disease, and brucellosis)

    b. *The Global Health Security Agenda (GHSA)*: Strengthens pandemic preparedness through One Health initiatives.

6. *Public awareness and community engagement* through public health education by veterinarians, environmental experts, and healthcare providers. For example, rabies control programs: Vaccination efforts in wildlife populations

2.2.2.3 Key components of one health surveillance in Europe

1. *Collaborative Frameworks and Agencies*: Like other countries, under the aegis of One Health approach, different organizations are working in unison in Europe too, such as

    a. *European Food Safety Authority (EFSA)*: It plays a pivotal role in monitoring zoonotic pathogens and providing risk assessments to support European Union (EU) legislation, such as Regulation (EU) 2016/429, which focuses on controlling the transmissibility of zoonotic diseases.

    b. *European Centre for Disease Prevention and Control (ECDC)*: ECDC emphasizes the importance of efforts to maintain integrity between humans, animals, and the environment.

2. *Coordinated surveillance and reporting*: Annual Zoonoses reports: EFSA and ECDC jointly publish comprehensive reports on zoonotic diseases within EU member states. For example, according to the report of the European Union one health in 2023, campylobacteriosis and salmonellosis remained the most reported zoonoses

3. *Regulatory and strategic initiatives*: To prevent antibiotic misuse and ensure the safety of the environment, several measures were implemented, such as

    a. *EU One Health Action Plan against Antimicrobial Resistance (AMR)*: To shut out the misuse of antimicrobials in human and veterinary medicine to combat AMR.

    b. *Farm to Fork Strategy (2020)*: This strategy was adopted for food safety purposes, incorporating One Health principles to ensure animal welfare and reduce disease transmission risks.

4. *Climate Change and Health Initiatives*: The European Climate and Health Observatory, launched in February 2021, centers on evaluating and handling the impacts of climate change on health [30].

2.3 Success stories

There are numerous examples across the world where the One Health approach has alleviated the dreaded effects of zoonotic diseases.

a. One such example is the substantial decrease in the mortality rate due to rabies in Sri Lanka, Bhutan, Bangladesh, and India (Jaipur, Sikkim, Chennai, and Goa), where the infections were uncontrollable before the One Health policy's execution. Active surveillance, expedited laboratory testing, strategic mass vaccination of dogs, pre-exposure (high-risk cases) and post-exposure vaccination in humans, and management of the dog population by Animal Birth Control (ABC Program) are the crucial steps in these areas to control rabies. In Bhutan, only 17 confirmed rabies cases were registered between 2006 and 2016, in Bangladesh, a notable reduction from 1500 deaths in 2006 to 200 deaths was observed, and in Sri Lanka, fewer than 50 deaths were reported in 2012 [31].

b. Another example is the successful containment of the Hendra virus in Australia by the development and vaccination of horses against the Hendra virus under the One Health approach through the Hendra surveillance system in horses [31].

c. Similarly, in the Arab countries, the One Health approach was of great help in the preparedness and alleviation of MERS-CoV cases. A workgroup was built in Qatar in 2015 in collaboration with the FAO, WHO, and OIE; representatives from the Middle East and Arab countries, along with health experts from all over the world, participated in the workshop, in which policies and strategic plans were designed and implemented for the restraints of MERS-CoV. According to the ECDC, as of 7 June 2023, no new MERS-CoV cases have been reported by any health authorities worldwide [31].

d. Previously taken as a mild disease until October 2015, when the Zika virus was associated with microcephaly cases in neonates in the maternity facilities of northeast Brazil. Up to December 2016, there were 174,667 confirmed cases, 528,157 suspected cases, and 18 Zika virus-related deaths reported, followed by the declaration by WHO that Zika virus infection was "a public health emergency of global concern". The outbreak was successfully tackled by executing the One Health concept: diagnostic tests, vaccine development, mosquito control, and public campaigns [31].

e. The Ebola virus outbreak in West Africa, 2014–2016 (The deadliest Ebola outbreak, with 28,000+ cases and 11,000+ deaths) and Uganda, 2022 (142 confirmed cases, 55 deaths, 39% fatality rate) was successfully controlled through One Health approach by the rapid diagnostic testing, strict handling protocols of deceased individuals and infected persons, vaccination, border health screening and community engagement [31].

f. In addition, the efforts to vaccinate children against DPT (diphtheria/tetanus/pertussis) and polio in Chad and the control measures for animals to prevent the spread of bovine pleuropneumonia contributed to a comprehensive coverage in both humans and animals [31].

g. In Kyrgyzstan, under the holistic One Health approach, public health professionals and veterinary people started working in collaboration, leading to a decrease in the economic loss related to echinococcosis, brucellosis, and other zoonotic diseases surveillance. In Canada, the adoption of the One Health approach led to a 26% reduction in overhead [31].

h. Lastly, the emergence of SARS-CoV-2 leading to the COVID-19 pandemic is a perfect example of a zoonotic pandemic. It was a modified virus of the Coronaviridae family of bat origin, with pangolins probably being the intermediate host that originated in the wet market of Wuhan, China, and transmitted to humans in late December 2019. In January 2020, the WHO declared it "a Public Health Emergency of International Concern." Finally, through strict adherence to the One Health approach through advanced diagnostic methods such as sequencing studies to know the variants and mutations, rapid vaccine development and mass immunization campaigns worldwide, lockdowns, social distancing, and masks helped in the reduction of transmission, and many countries restricted wet markets and illegal wildlife trade to prevent future zoonotic spillovers resulted in constraints of the pandemic [31].

A few significant success stories of different countries are depicted in **Table 1.**

Name of the disease or pathogen contained/controlled	Name of the country/continent	Approach under the One Health policy
Rabies	Sri Lanka, Bhutan, Bangladesh, and India (Jaipur, Sikkim, Chennai, and Goa)	• Active surveillance • Expedited laboratory testing, strategic mass vaccination of dogs • Pre-exposure (high-risk cases) and post-exposure vaccination in humans • Animal Birth Control (ABC Program) - control dog population
MERS-CoV	Arab countries	• The workgroup to restraint MERS-CoV was built in Qatar in collaboration with the FAO, WHO, and OIE • Various workshops and training programs are conducted to design strategic plans and implement policies
Hendra virus	Australia	• Development and vaccination of horses against the Hendra virus
ZIKV	Brazil	• Prompt diagnostic tests • Vaccine development • Mosquito control measures • Public campaigns
EVD	West Africa, Uganda	• Rapid diagnostic testing • Strict handling protocols of deceased individuals and infected persons • Vaccination • Border health screening and community engagement
SARS-CoV-2; COVID-19 pandemic	Worldwide	• Advanced diagnostic methods (sequencing) • Rapid vaccine development • Mass immunization campaigns • Worldwide lockdowns, social distancing, and the use of masks • Restrictions on wet markets and illegal wildlife trade

Note: MERS-CoV – middle east respiratory syndrome coronavirus, ZIKV - zika virus, EVD - Ebola virus disease, SARS-CoV-2 – severe acute respiratory syndrome coronavirus 2, COVID-19 – coronavirus disease 19.

Table 1.
Country/continent-wise success stories under the aegis of the One Health approach.

2.4 Lessons learned from one health approach in zoonotic disease control and critical analysis of key success factors

From several experiences of incidences of various infectious diseases across the globe, researchers, stakeholders, policy makers, and the inhabitants have learned the following lessons:

1. Active zoonotic disease surveillance in wildlife is crucial for outbreak prediction.
2. Zoonotic spillover risks must be addressed at the point of origin (wildlife trade and deforestation).
3. Intersectoral collaborations in the multiple dimensions, like public and animal, and environmental sectors, ensure an effective response.
4. Rapid diagnostic testing, identification, vaccination, and containment can prevent large-scale outbreaks.
5. Border health screening is essential to prevent cross-country spread.
6. Vigilant monitoring in wet markets can prevent human infections.
7. Effective poultry vaccinations can help reduce the risk of spillover to humans.
8. Rabies is 100% preventable with effective vaccination
9. Community engagement and awareness campaigns are critical to control the spread of zoonotic diseases.
10. Global cooperation is essential for pandemic preparedness, and substantial investment in One Health activities can prevent future pandemics.

2.4.1 Critical analysis of key success factors

- *Integrated Surveillance & Early Detection*: Rapid diagnostic testing and coordinated surveillance systems (e.g., rabies, MERS-CoV, and Ebola) facilitated timely intervention and containment.
- *Mass Vaccination Programs*: Systematic immunization campaigns (rabies, Hendra virus, Ebola, DPT, and polio) significantly reduced mortality rates and infection spread.
- *Vector and Reservoir Management*: Targeted interventions, such as mosquito control (zika virus) and dog population management (rabies), minimized transmission risks.
- *Community Engagement and Public Awareness*: Public health education campaigns enhanced compliance, reduced stigma, and improved disease prevention, especially in Ebola and COVID-19 responses.

- *Policy and Strategic Implementation*: Government-led initiatives backed by international agencies ensured structured execution, which is evident in MERS-CoV containment.

2.5 Future directions

The One Health approach is increasingly recognized as a core feature for managing zoonotic diseases. Future directions emphasize more robust partnerships across different sectors to effectively mitigate these diseases. For the successful accomplishment of the goals, various steps need to be taken and implemented, such as strengthening intersectoral collaborations, aligning policies across sectors to facilitate joint planning and resource allocation, developing unified platforms that consolidate data from human, animal, and environmental health sectors which in turn enhance early detection and timely response to zoonotic diseases. Furthermore, the design and development of curricula emphasizing integrated approaches to health can prepare future professionals for collaborative work, conducting training programs and workshops that ensure that current professionals stay vigilant for any of the emerging threats. In addition to it, to achieve sustainable land management, effective land-use practices should be implemented to preserve biodiversity and reduce human-wildlife contact to lower the risks of zoonotic disease transmission, and different laws and policies should be enforced to address and alleviate the climate change issues responsible for the zoonotic disease spillover [13, 30, 31].

3. Conclusion

The One Health approach provides a sustainable, integrated framework for combating infectious diseases, emphasizing long-term solutions and global collaboration. In an interconnected world, no single nation or discipline can confront resurging pathogens alone. Strengthening cross-sectoral partnerships among human, animal, and environmental health professionals is essential for transformative breakthroughs and accelerated innovations. Ensuring sustainable funding for interdisciplinary research supports advancements in diagnostics, surveillance, and intervention strategies, while establishing international policies enhances global health security. Equally important is empowering communities and local stakeholders with scientific knowledge and practical interventions through education and engagement, ensuring effective disease prevention and response. Protecting ecosystem integrity by regulating wildlife trade and addressing environmental drivers of zoonotic spillovers remains a critical component of One Health strategies. Through unified global efforts, the One Health framework safeguards health across species and paves the path for a future prepared to tackle emerging infectious threats.

Author details

Monalisa Mohanty[1], Sutapa Rath[2], Gayatree Nayak[3]*, Preetam Kumar Kar[4] and Jeebanjyoti Mishra[5]

1 Department of Microbiology, IMS & SUM Hospital, Bhubaneswar, India

2 Yashoda Hospital, Hitech City, Hyderabad, India

3 Department of Microbiology, KIMS, Bhubaneswar, India

4 Department of Community Medicine, SCB Medical College and Hospital, Cuttack, India

5 Department of Dermatology, KIMS, Bhubaneswar, India

*Address all correspondence to: gayatreenayak02@gmail.com

References

[1] One Health High Level Expert Panel. Geneva, Switzerland: World Health Organization; 2023. Available from: https://www.who. int/publications/m/item/one-health-definitions-and-principles [Accessed: April 15, 2025]

[2] One Health Initiative Task Force (OHITF). One Health: A New Professional Imperative. Schaumburg, Illinois, USA: American Veterinary Medical Association (AVMA); 2008. Available from: https://www.avma.org/sites/default/fles/resources/onehealth_fnal.pdf

[3] Wang S, Li W, Wang Z, Yang W, et al. Emerging and reemerging infectious diseases: Global trends and new strategies for their prevention and control. Signal Transduction and Targeted Therapy. 2024;**9**(1):223. DOI: 10.1038/s41392-024-01917-x

[4] Mehand MS, Al-Shorbaji F, Millett P, Murgue B. The WHO R&D blueprint: 2018 review of emerging infectious diseases requiring urgent research and development efforts. Antiviral Research. 2018;**159**:63-67. DOI: 10.1016/j.antiviral.2018.09.009

[5] Roncada P, Modesti A, Timperio AM, et al. One medicine–one health–one biology and many proteins: Proteomics on the verge of the one health approach. Molecular BioSystems. 2014;**10**(6):1226-1227. DOI: 10.1039/c4mb90011a

[6] Sasidharan S, Standley CJ. One health, one future: A unified approach to a balanced ecosystem. Tropical Medicine and Infectious Disease. 2024;**9**(7):164. DOI: 10.3390/tropicalmed9070164

[7] Lerner H. Philosophical roots of the one medicine movement: An analysis of some relevant ideas by Rudolf Virchow and Calvin Schwabe with their modern implications. SPE. 2013;**6**:97-109. DOI: 10.12697/spe.2013.6.2.07

[8] Pitt SJ, Gunn A. The one health concept. British Journal of Biomedical Science. 2024;**81**:12366. DOI: 10.3389/bjbs.2024.12366

[9] Mackenzie JS et al. One Health: The Human-Animal-Environment Interfaces in Emerging Infectious Diseases. 1st ed. Heidelberg: Springer; 2013

[10] Sinclair JR. Importance of a one health approach in advancing global health security and the sustainable development goals. Revue Scientifique et Technique. 2019;**38**(1):145-154. DOI: 10.20506/rst.38.1.2949

[11] Food and Agriculture Organization of the United Nations (FAO). Taking a Multisectoral, One Health Approach: A Tripartite Guide to Addressing Zoonotic Diseases in Countries. Rome, Italy, Paris, France, Geneva, Switzerland: Food and Agriculture Organization of the United Nations (FAO), World Organisation for Animal Health (OIE) & World Health Organization (WHO); 2019. 166 pp. Available from: www.oie.int/fileadmin/Home/eng/Media_Center/docs/EN_TripartiteZoonosesGuide_web.pdf

[12] FAO, UNEP, WHO, and WOAH. One Health Joint Plan of Action (2022-2026). Working Together for the Health of Humans, Animals, Plants and the Environment. Rome, Italy: Food and Agriculture Organization of the United Nations (FAO), United Nations Environment Programme(UNEP), World Health Organization (WHO), World Organisation For Animal Health (WOAH); 2022. DOI: 10.4060/cc2289en

[13] Mishra B, Rath S, Mohanty M, Mohapatra PR. The threat of impending pandemics: A proactive approach. Cureus. 2023;**15**(3):e36723. DOI: 10.7759/cureus.36723

[14] Mazet JA, Uhart MM, Keyyu JD. Stakeholders in one health. Revue Scientifique et Technique. 2014;**33**(2):443-452. DOI: 10.20506/rst.33.2.2295

[15] Erkyihun GA, Alemayehu MB. One health approach for the control of zoonotic diseases. Zoonoses. 2022;**2**(1):963. DOI: 10.15212/ZOONOSES-2022-0037

[16] Asaaga FA, Young JC, Oommen MA, et al. Operationalising the "one health" approach in India: Facilitators of and barriers to effective cross-sector convergence for zoonoses prevention and control. BMC Public Health. 2021;**21**(1):1517. DOI: 10.1186/s12889-021-11545-7

[17] Dar OA, Akhbari M, Nacer H. Multisectoral one health collaborations across human, animal and environmental health: A protocol paper for an umbrella systematic review of conceptual and analytical approaches to sustainability. BMJ Open. 2024;**14**(12):e086248. DOI: 10.1136/bmjopen-2024-086248

[18] Hegewisch-Taylor J, Dreser A, Aragón-Gama AC, et al. One health governance and implementation challenges in Mexico. Global Public Health. 2024;**19**(1):2377259. DOI: 10.1080/17441692.2024.2377259

[19] Yopa DS, Massom DM, Kiki GM, et al. Barriers and enablers to the implementation of one health strategies in developing countries: A systematic review. Frontiers in Public Health. 2023;**11**:1252428. DOI: 10.3389/fpubh.2023.1252428

[20] Hayman DTS, Adisasmito WB, Almuhairi S, et al. Developing one health surveillance systems. One Health. 2023;**17**:100617. DOI: 10.1016/j.onehlt.2023.100617

[21] Milazzo A, Liu J, Multani P, Steele S, Hoon E, Chaber AL. One health implementation: A systematic scoping review using the quadripartite one health joint plan of action. One Health. 2025;**20**:101008. DOI: 10.1016/j.onehlt.2025.101008

[22] Ghanbari MK, Gorji HA, Behzadifar M, Shoghli A, Martini M. Strategic planning, components and evolution in zoonotic diseases frameworks: One health approach and public health ethics. Journal of Preventive Medicine and Hygiene. 2022;**62**(4):E981-E987. DOI: 10.15167/2421-4248/jpmh2021.62.4.2323

[23] Sun ZS, Wan EY, Agbana YL, et al. Global one health index for zoonoses: A performance assessment in 160 countries and territories. iScience. 2024;**27**(4):109297. DOI: 10.1016/j.isci.2024.109297

[24] Food and Agriculture Organization of the United Nations (FAO), World Organisation for Animal Health (WOAH, formerly OIE), World Health Organization (WHO). Taking a Multisectoral One Health Approach: A Tripartite Guide to Addressing Zoonotic Diseases in Countries [Internet]. Rome, Italy: Food and Agriculture Organization of the United Nations (FAO); 2019. Available from: https://www.fao.org/one-health/resources/publications/guide-to-addressing-zoonotic-diseases-in-countries/ [Accessed: April 16, 2025]

[25] National Center for Emerging and Zoonotic Infectious Diseases (NCEZID), a division of the CDC. One Health

in Action Stories [Internet]. Atlanta, Georgia, USA: Centers for Disease Control and Prevention (CDC); 2023. Available from: https://www.cdc.gov/one-health/php/stories/index.html [Accessed: April 16, 2025]

[26] Tangwangvivat R, Rungsitiyakorn R, Hoonaukit C, et al. Collective activities of the Thai coordinating unit for one health (CUOH): Past activities and future directions. One Health. 2024;**18**:100728. DOI: 10.1016/j.onehlt.2024.100728

[27] Innes GK, Lambrou AS, Thumrin P, Thukngamdee Y, Tangwangvivat R, Doungngern P, et al. Enhancing global health security in Thailand: Strengths and challenges of initiating a one health approach to avian influenza surveillance. One Health. 2022;**14**:100397. DOI: 10.1016/j.onehlt.2022.100397

[28] Krishnasamy V, Behravesh CB, Varela K, Goryoka G, Oussayef N, Rooney J, et al. 677. Using a multisectoral one health approach to prioritize zoonotic diseases in the United States. Open Forum Infectious Diseases. 2018;**5**(Suppl. 1):S244. DOI: 10.1093/ofid/ofy210.683

[29] U.S. One Health Coordination Unit (U.S. OHCU). National One Health Framework to Address Zoonotic Diseases and Advance Public Health Preparedness in the United States. [Internet]. Atlanta, Georgia, USA: Centers for Disease Control and Prevention (CDC); 2025. Available from: https://www.cdc.gov/one-health/media/pdfs/2025/01/354391-A-NOHF-ZOONOSES-508_FINAL.pdf [Accessed: April 18, 2025]

[30] European Food Safety Authority (EFSA), Berezowski J, de Balogh K, Dórea FC, et al. Prioritisation of zoonotic diseases for coordinated surveillance systems under the one health approach for cross-border pathogens that threaten the union. EFSA Journal. 2023;**21**(3):e07853. DOI: 10.2903/j.efsa.2023.7853

[31] Horefti E. The importance of the one health concept in combating Zoonoses. Pathogens. 2023;**12**(8):977. DOI: 10.3390/pathogens12080977

Chapter 3

Arboviruses: Dynamics of Infection and Immune Evasion during the Replication Cycles

Manuel Alejandro Mosso Pani, Henry Puerta-Guardo, Daniel Nunez-Avellaneda, Nicole M. Nazario Maldonado and Luis Antonio Alonso-Palomares

Abstract

Arboviruses (arthropod-borne viruses) are etiological viral agents mainly transmitted by arthropod vectors that pose a significant burden on the human public health systems worldwide, causing millions of infections every year; these viruses need to replicate in hematophagous arthropods, including numerous species of mosquitoes, ticks, and midges, among others. Important arboviruses for human and animal health include the dengue virus (DENV), Mayaro virus (MAYV), Rift Valley fever virus (RVFV), Zika virus (ZIKV), Yellow fever virus (YFV), chikungunya (CHIKV), and African swine fever virus (ASF), among other closely related viruses. These infectious agents can infect different hosts (invertebrate vectors and mammalian hosts), which requires avoiding two types of immune responses to continue and remain in nature. Arboviruses have sylvatic (vector to wild animals) and urban (vector to humans) transmission cycles and have developed mechanisms to overcome ecological and biological challenges, allowing them to take over the cellular machinery and successfully complete their replication cycle among hosts. Despite numerous pieces of evidence and studies, the mechanisms, molecules, and components involved in the arbovirus replication cycles are yet to be defined. This chapter will discuss viral replication processes, immune evasion, and vaccine development for arboviral families that are relevant to public health.

Keywords: arbovirus, replication cycle, immune evasion, vector-borne viruses, Flaviviridae, Togaviridae, Reoviridae, Asfaviridae, Bunyaviridae

1. Introduction

Arboviruses are viruses transmitted by arthropod vectors to vertebrate hosts during blood-feeding and can involve animal reservoirs. Globally, an estimated 2.5 million deaths are recorded annually, making vector-borne diseases a serious and growing public health burden. Arboviruses predominate in tropical and subtropical countries and are closely related to the vector distribution [1]. Recently, there has been a concerning rise in the spread of several arboviruses, along with the emergence of new transmission cycles. Additionally, these viruses might adapt to new vectors and change environmental conditions [2].

Most of these viruses are primarily transmitted by mosquitoes and ticks as vectors. However, not all species can transmit all viruses. This ability depends on several factors, including molecular mechanisms, adaptability, dissemination, immune response evasion, and transmission dynamics involving the pathogen, the vector, and the mammalian host. Additionally, all of these processes are affected by external factors, which can be biotic and abiotic [2]. Furthermore, other arthropod species, such as midges (e.g., Family *Ceratopogonidae*; genus *Culicoides*), have recently gained increased attention due to the imminent threat of transmitting viruses, especially those belonging to the genus *Orthobunyavirus* [3].

Over 100 species of arboviruses that cause diseases in humans have been identified. Their classification may vary, but the following families are typically included: *Bunyaviridae, Flaviviridae, Reoviridae, Asfaviridae, and Togaviridae* (**Table 1**).

Vector ecology is crucial for the adaptability, survival, establishment, and transmission of arboviruses in nature. Arboviral transmission encompasses four primary cycles: (1) sylvatic, which involves transmission from vectors to wild animals such as birds and primates; (2) urban, where transmission occurs from vectors to humans; (3) epizootic, involving transmission from vectors to domestic animals like pigs and horses; and (4) zoonotic, which involves transmission from vectors to animals, followed by transmission from infected animals to humans. The vector acquires the infectious agent from an infected mammal host through blood-feeding, a process known as horizontal transmission (spreading disease between individuals in the same population). Following this, the vector undergoes an extrinsic incubation period (EIP). This is the time it takes for the mosquito to become infected after the viral replication has started. During this period, the virus spreads to various tissues, including the salivary glands. The virus can then be transmitted to another host through saliva during a second blood meal, thus completing the transmission cycle. Additionally, numerous studies have demonstrated that transovarial transmission (vertical) plays a significant role in passing these viruses to the next generation and remains in nature [4].

Arboviruses can infect both invertebrates and mammals. However, the successful establishment of the infection requires effective invasion mechanisms that can overcome two types of immune systems: that of the arthropod (the carrier) and the mammal (the host). In invertebrate infections, pathogens must evade the innate immune system, which includes different defenses such as phagocytosis, reactive oxygen species (ROS), phenoloxidase (PO), myelinization, antimicrobial peptides, and several signaling pathways (Toll, immune deficiency pathway (IMD), Janus kinase-signal transducer and activator of transcription (JAK-STAT), and RNA interference (RNAi)). Evidence suggests that invertebrates possess thioester-containing proteins (TEPs) similar to the C3 complement protein in vertebrates. These proteins assist in the opsonization and elimination of pathogens [5]. In humans, arboviruses encounter multiple components of the immune system. This includes the innate immune system, which comprises dendritic cells (DC), macrophages, and neutrophils, as well as key molecules like cytokines and interferons (IFNs). Additionally, these viruses must contend with the adaptive immune system, which consists of antibodies and memory cells (B and T cells). By understanding and researching the different stages of viral replication within host cells, we can create strategies to mitigate the negative impacts of these diseases. These illnesses have posed significant challenges to the food industry and public health globally, affecting millions of people.

Family	Genome	Virus examples	Site of replication	Main vector	Other vectors	Host
Flaviviridae	(+) ssRNA Linear	Dengue	Cytoplasm	*Ae. aegypti* *Ae. albopictus*	Other species within the Aedes spp.	Human nonhuman primates, pigs, marsupials, bats, birds, horses, bovid, rodents, and dogs
		Zika	Cytoplasm	*Ae. aegypti* *Ae. albopictus*	*Ae. hensilii*	Human and nonhuman primates
		Yellow fever	Cytoplasm	*Ae. aegypti*	*Haemagogus* and *Sabethes spp.*	Human and nonhuman primates
		West Nile	Cytoplasm	*Cx. pipiens*	*Ae. rusticus* *Ae. albopictus*	Birds and human
		Japanese encephalitis	Cytoplasm	*Cx. tritaeniorhynchus*	*Ae. albopictus* and *Cx. quinquefasciatus*	Human and nonhuman primates, pigs, birds
Togaviridae	(+) ssRNA	Chikungunya	Cytoplasm	*Ae. aegypti*		Human
		Mayaro	Cytoplasm	*Ae. aegypti*	*An. freeborni* *An. gambiae* *An. stephensi*	Human
		Venezuelan equine encephalitis	Cytoplasm	*Cx. tarsalis*		Human
Reoviridae	(+) dsRNA	Bluetongue	Cytoplasm	*Culicoides tainanus*	*Culicoides tainanus* and *Culicoides cryptic*	Cattle and sheep
		Colorado tick fever virus	Cytoplasm	*Dermacentor andersoni, Dermacentor variabilis* and *Rhipicephalus sanguineus*	*Dermancentor variabilis* and *Rhipicephalus sanguineus*	Squirrels, chipmunk, and mice
Asfaviridae	dsDNA	African swine fever virus	Cytoplasm	*Ornithodoros moubata porcinus*		Domestic pigs, warthogs, wild boars, and bush pigs
				Ornithodoros moubata		

Family	Genome	Virus examples	Site of replication	Main vector	Other vectors	Host
Bunyaviridae	(−) ssRNA	La Crosse encephalitis virus	*Cytoplasm/ Nucleus*	*Aedes triseriatus*	*Ae. albopictus* and *Ae. aegypti*	Humans
		Congo hemorrhagic fever virus	*Cytoplasm/ Nucleus*	Species within the *Hyalomma* genus	*Hyalomma rufipes, Hyalomma Truncatum, Amblyomma variegatum, Rhipicephalus evertsi evertsi, Rhipicephalus appendiculatus, and Dermacentor marginatus*	Humans, water buffalo, goats, sheep, cattle, hares, African hedgehogs, and mice
		Rift Valley fever virus	*Cytoplasm/ Nucleus*	*Aedes spp*	*Culex, Mansonia,* and *Anopheles*	Humans, cattle, sheep, and goats

Table 1.
Arboviruses and their vectors: Viruses and their vectors are grouped by genus and genomic characteristics of each family. Aedes (Ae.), Culex (Cx).

2. *Flaviviridae:* General features, replication cycle, and immune evasion strategies

The *Flaviviridae* family comprises several enveloped viruses with a positive-sense single-stranded ribonucleic acid (+ssRNA), including the DENV, YFV, ZIKV, West Nile virus (WNV), tick-borne encephalitis virus (TBE), and Japanese encephalitis virus (JEV) (**Table 1**). These viruses contain a single open reading frame (ORF) that encodes the polyprotein, flanked by two untranslated regions (UTRs), one at the 5′ and the other at the 3′ terminus. Mosquitoes transmit these arboviruses, and they can cause a range of symptoms, from mild to severe, potentially leading to life-threatening outcomes like hemorrhages. Additionally, individuals who have been infected may experience the development of encephalitis and other severe neurological conditions. ZIKV has been linked to congenital disabilities, particularly microcephaly, which the mother can acquire during pregnancy. The only vaccine available from this family is for the YFV, which is recommended for travelers visiting endemic areas. Studying the replicative cycle of *Flaviviridae* viruses can help identify targets for antiviral drugs and vaccine design [6].

The *Flaviviridae* virus initiates the viral replicative cycle by attaching its envelope protein to specific cellular receptors on the host cell surface (**Figure 1**). The receptors required may differ depending on the flavivirus and host cell type. After binding to the cell surface, the virus is endocytosed by a clathrin-dependent mechanism [7]. In an

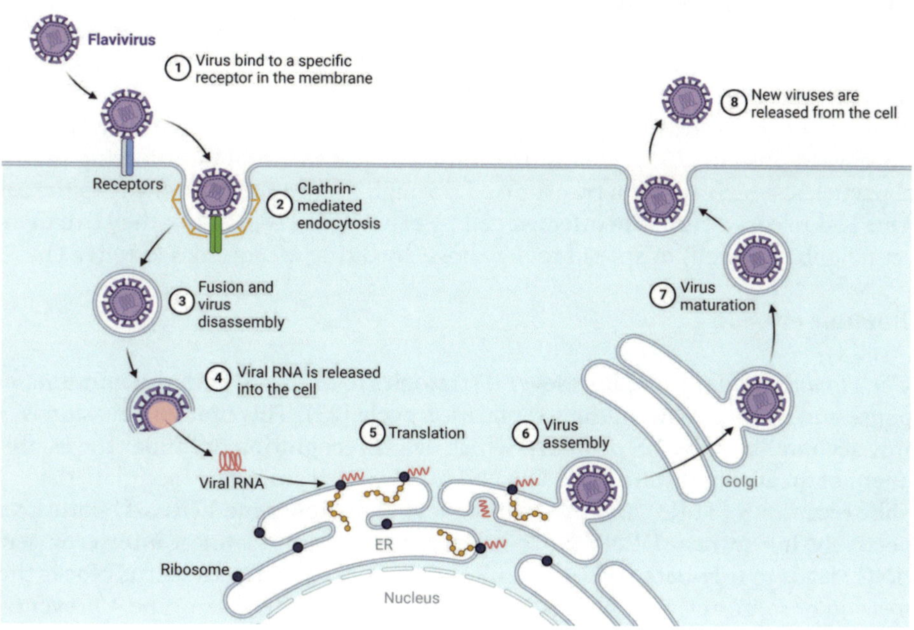

Figure 1.
Schematic representation of the Flaviviridae *virus replicative cycle. The cycle begins with the virus attaching through the envelope protein (E) to specific cellular receptors on the host cell. Subsequent steps include endocytosis, where the virus is internalized through a clathrin-dependent mechanism, and membrane fusion, characterized by a conformational change in viral envelope proteins that facilitates fusion with the endosomal membrane. Following these initial stages, host ribosomes utilize viral RNA as a template for translation, synthesizing a polyprotein. The viral RNA also serves as a template for replication. The final stage involves the assembly of viral components to form mature virions. These mature virions are eventually released from the infected cell through exocytosis, allowing them to spread to new hosts, often transmitted through mosquito bites.*

environment with low pH, the viral envelope proteins facilitate the fusion of the viral and endosomal membranes through a conformational change [8]. This fusion allows the release of the viral genome into the cytoplasm of the host cell [9]. Ribosomes use the viral RNA as a template for translation; this results in the production of a large polyprotein that contains a structural capsid (C), precursor membrane (prM), envelope (E), and seven nonstructural (NS1, NS2A, NS2B, NS3, NS4A, NS4B, and NS5) proteins [10]. The NS proteins play essential roles in viral replication and evasion of the host immune system [11]. The viral RNA genome is then used as a template for the replication and transcription process. The RNA-dependent RNA polymerase (RdRp) encoded in the viral genome produces negative-strand RNA, which is used as a replicative intermediate for synthesizing new positive-sense RNA genomes [12].

Furthermore, the virus encodes its structural proteins (SP) by transcribing shorter subgenomic RNA molecules [12, 13]. After the new positive-sense RNA genomes are synthesized, the SP accumulate in the endoplasmic reticulum (ER). Some cytoplasmic viral proteins, such as C, NS1, and NS5 proteins, can be translocated to the nucleus during infection by DENV and ZIKV in mammal cells. Additionally, in mosquito cells (*Ae. albopictus)* infected with DENV, proteins like C, NS1, NS3, and NS5 have been observed in the nucleus [14, 15]. Although little is known about the role of these proteins in this compartment, mutations in nuclear-signaling proteins such as C and NS5 cause a reduction in viral replication [16, 17]. It has recently been shown that the NS3 protein of DENV and ZIKV hijacks the function of the nuclear pore complex and controls nuclear-cytoplasmic transport [15, 18]. Viral genome replication and assembly are closely associated with specialized membrane structures called viral replication complexes [19]. C proteins encapsulate the new RNA genomes to form the nucleocapsid, which attaches to the ER lumen and acquires a bilipid membrane from the ER membrane that contains viral glycoproteins, including the E and prM proteins. The prM is cleaved by host cell proteases in the secretory pathway, forming the mature M protein [20, 21]. This maturation step is essential for infecting new viral particles, which are then transported through the secretory pathway to the cell surface and released from the infected cell by exocytosis [14, 15, 22]; they can then infect neighboring cells or spread to new hosts by biting mosquitoes (**Figure 1**).

2.1 Immune evasion

The Flavivirus family employs several strategies to interfere with the immune response and be successful in their replication cycle [23]. This immune evasion is mainly accomplished by NS proteins, which evade recognition or hinder the establishment of an antiviral state [24]. The NS1 and NS2A from WNV modulate the toll-like receptor 3 (TLR3) and the retinoic acid-inducible gene 1 (RIG-I) pathways, respectively. In contrast, DENV NS2B3 cleavage of the stimulator of interferon genes (STING) leads to IFN-beta (IFN-β) suppression. Subsequently, the virus blocks the expression of some antiviral molecules; the NS4B from DENV serotype 4 prevents the IFN production, blocking the phosphorylation of the signal transducer and activator of transcription (STAT). Ultimately, the virus neutralizes the functional activity of these antiviral molecules [11]. Additionally, activated innate immune pathways, including complement, apoptosis, and autophagy, can be evaded or exploited by the virus to exacerbate the disease [24]. Although the NS and SP of *Flavivirus* contribute significantly to immune evasion, the specific targets are still undisclosed. How these proteins collaborate to weaken the innate immune system is currently unknown. Further research is necessary to develop new vaccines for flaviviruses, including those currently available in some countries, to understand their immune evasion tactics better and identify potential target areas.

3. *Togaviridae:* General features, replication cycle, and immune evasion strategies

Togaviruses belonging to the *Alphavirus* genus include CHIKV, MAYV, Sindbis virus (SINV), and western equine encephalitis virus (WEEV). The *Alphavirus* genus has a positive-sense single-stranded RNA (+ssRNA) genome (**Table 1**). Its genome size typically measures around 12 kb, and it contains two open reading frames (ORFs) that encode SP and NS, both of which are separated by a noncoding sequence [25]. A short code for the four nonstructural proteins (nsP 1–4) is generated from the cleavage of the polyprotein. nsP1 is involved in RNA capping, nsP2 has helicase and protease activities, and nsP3 contains three recognized domains (the macro domain, the alphavirus unique domain (AUD), and the hypervariable region), all of which are required for viral replication. The nsP4 protein is responsible for RNA synthesis and functions as an RdRp. The SP generate several components essential for the virus's structure. It produces the C protein, the E glycoproteins E1, E2, and E3, and the 6 K protein, which interacts with the E1 and E2 proteins. Additionally, it produces the transframe protein (TF), which plays a role in viral assembly [26, 27].

Many of the replication processes and the possible role of viral proteins during the infection are still unknown; many of the functions of these proteins are inferred from some *alphaviruses*, such as CHIKV. The virus binds to the target cell receptor using the E2 protein; some receptors have been characterized, such as the matrix remodeling associate 8 (Mxra8) molecule (also known as DICAM or ASP3), which is used to endocytose the MAYV [28]. The cell takes up the viral particle through endocytosis, leading to the formation of an endosome. As the endosome becomes more acidic, the envelope proteins undergo structural changes, exposing the E1 protein. This exposure promotes the fusion of the virus with the cell membrane, releasing the nucleocapsid and the viral genome into the cell. Afterward, the viral genome is synthesized into nsP precursors from the viral mRNA. The nsP produces a replication complex (RC) too. The RC facilitates the synthesis of the negative RNA strand, which serves as a template for producing the genomic (49S) and subgenomic (26S) RNA. The 26S subgenomic RNA is used to produce a structural polyprotein. The nucleocapsid is assembled when the capsid protein surrounds the 49S genomic RNA through the action of serine proteases. The maturation of the E1 and E2 glycoproteins occurs in the ER and Golgi complex. This maturation is directly linked to the transport and release of new viral particles at the cell membrane (**Figure 2**) [29].

These viruses are transmitted by arthropod vectors, specifically by mosquito species such as *Ae. aegypti*, *Ae. albopictus*, and *Culex spp.* These mosquitoes inject saliva and introduce the viral particles into the host bloodstream while taking away blood, which is necessary to provide nutrients for the subsequent progeny. Studies have found that a mutation in protein E2 of a CHIKV genotype increases susceptibility and transmission in *Aedes albopictus* mosquitoes [30].

3.1 Immune evasion

Most alphaviruses produce similar symptoms in humans, including fever, rash, headache, eye pain, muscle pain, conjunctivitis, and joint pain. These symptoms can

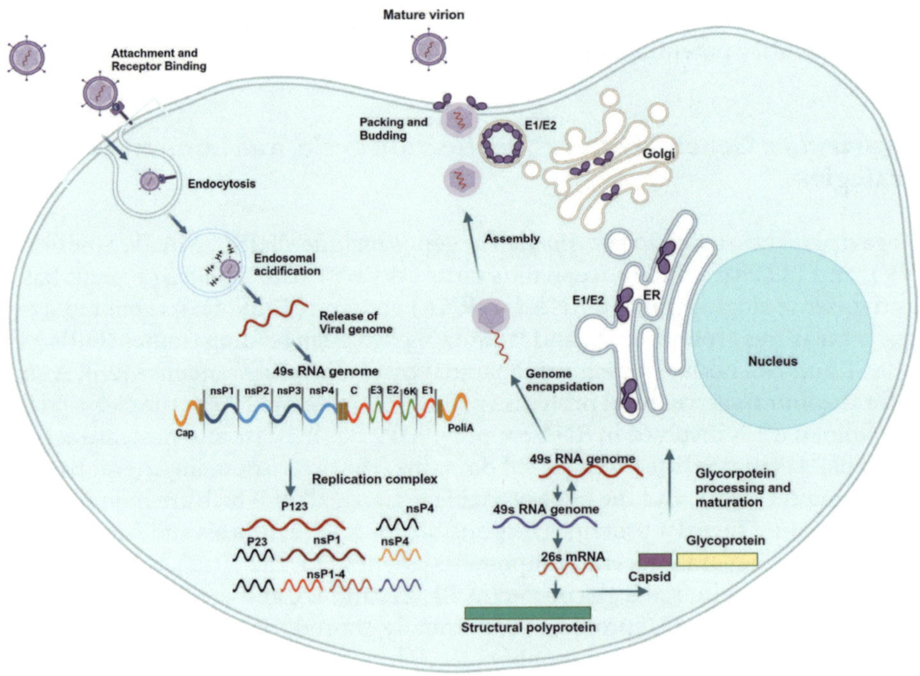

Figure 2.
Schematic representation of the replication cycle of the Togaviridae*. The virus binds to host cell receptors and enters* via *endocytosis. Acidification of the endosome triggers the release of the viral genome into the cytoplasm. The RdRp produces viral replication complexes in the cytoplasm that generate 49 s and 29 s subgenomes. The 29S subgenome encodes the viral SP, while the 49S subgenome contains the genetic material necessary for packaging into the capsid. The Golgi complex assembles and matures glycoproteins E1 and E2. The mature virion will be released through the exocytosis of the cell itself.*

persist for months or even years, often leading to significant disability. Additionally, severe complications, such as neurological issues, myocarditis, and hemorrhagic manifestations, can occur as a result of the disease. This severity is linked to increased pro-inflammatory mediators and cytokines, including the monocyte chemoattractant protein-1 (MCP-1), interleukins (IL)-9, IL-13, Vascular endothelial growth factor (VEGF), IL-17, and interferon gamma-induced protein 10 (IP-10). Additionally, various other components are activated and released during the infection process. These include oxidative stress, apoptosis, TNF-α secretion, and ROS [31].

Several types of vaccines are in development, including attenuated viruses, RNA vaccines, and viral vectors. However, no effective vaccine has yet been approved for use. While some drugs are being evaluated, the most effective measures against diseases are treating symptoms and controlling the vector population.

4. *Reoviridae:* General features, replication cycle, and immune evasion strategies

The first mammalian reovirus identified in humans was an orthoreovirus. In the late 1950s, virions were found in the feces of children with gastrointestinal disease. The family includes 15 genera (Aquareovirus, Cardoreovirus, Coltivirus, Cypovirus, Fijivirus, Dinovernavirus, Idnoreovirus, Mimoreovirus, Mycoreovirus, Orbivirus, Orthoreovirus, Oryzavirus, Phytoreovirus, Rotavirus, and Seadornavirus) [32].

The family members possess a linear positive-sense double-stranded RNA (+dsRNA) molecule that is segmented, containing 9–12 segments. The viruses are non-enveloped. Viruses consist of two concentric protein shells: an outer capsid and an inner core that contains a genome of dsRNA segments. The virion has an icosahedral shape and ranges in size from 60 to 90 nm in diameter (**Figure 3**) [33, 34].

The process of viral replication takes place in the cytoplasm of host cells. After a virus enters a cell, its outer capsid is broken down by proteolytic cleavage in the late endosomes, forming transcriptionally active cores. This process triggers the synthesis of viral mRNA, which is then extruded for translation. Subsequently, cellular morphogenesis is guided by nsP. The NS1 protein enhances the translation of Bluetongue virus (BTV) ssRNA and facilitates the formation of tubules within the cytosol. Meanwhile, the NS2 protein produces viral inclusion bodies (VIBs), which concentrate viral proteins and newly synthesized ssRNAs for core assembly. After the cores are assembled and released from the VIBs, they are transported via endocytic vesicles through the interaction of NS3 with annexin and calpactin. Complete viral particles are formed when the core interacts with VP5 and VP2 during virion maturation. During the early stages of infection, virions exit the host cell non-lytically by utilizing the interaction between the NS3 protein and Tsg101. New viral particles are released before cell lysis occurs (**Figure 3**) [23, 24].

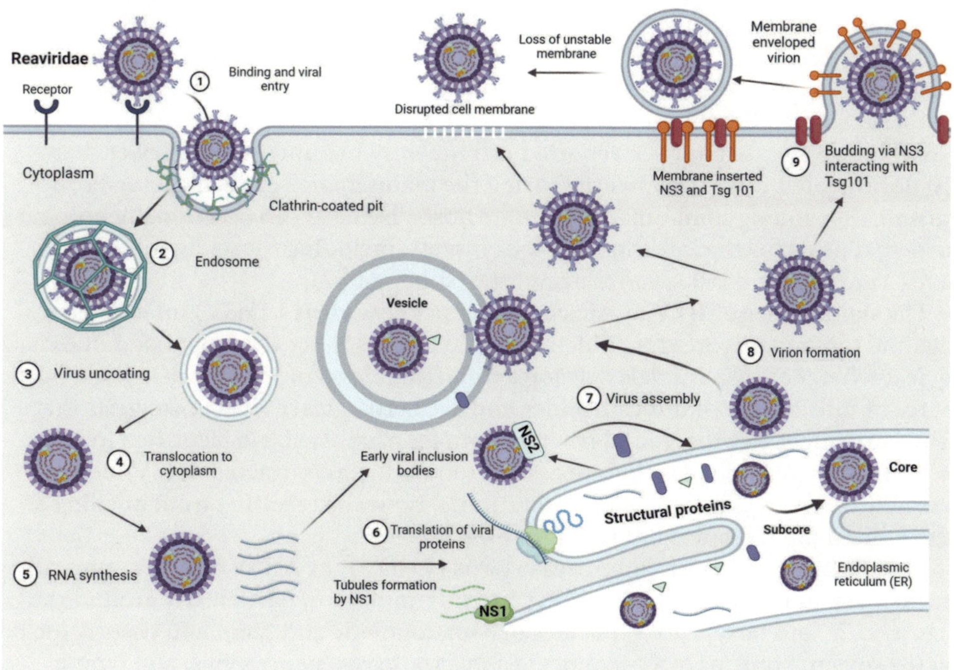

Figure 3.
Schematic representation of the Reoviridae family *replication cycle. (1–2) The virus attaches to the host receptor through glycoprotein and is endocytosed into clathrin-coated vesicles (3–4). The virus is uncoating, and the material genome is released in the cytoplasm. (5) NS1 promotes ssRNA translation (6) and subsequently forms tubules in the cytosol. (7) NS2 creates viral inclusion bodies that concentrate viral proteins and newly synthesized ssRNAs for core assembly. (8) Complete particles are formed when the core associates with VP5 and VP2, initiating the virion maturation. (9) During the early stages of infection, virions exit the cell non-lytically through NS3 interacting with Tsg101, leading to budding and eventual release without cell lysis.*

4.1 Arboviruses within the *Reoviridae* family

4.1.1 Coltiviruses

Coltiviruses are a type of virus belonging to the Spinovirinae subfamily. Recently discovered tick-borne viruses include the Colorado tick fever virus (CTFV), Eyach virus [35], Kundal virus [36], Tai forest reovirus [37], and Tarumizu tick virus [38]. Several coltiviruses have been named based on their nucleotide and protein sequences in the International Nucleotide Sequence Database Collaboration (INSDC). These include the California hare coltivirus, Gierle tick virus, Jeddah tick coltivirus, Salmon River virus, and Zeboroti virus. However, they are currently unclassified [39]. Coltiviruses contain 12 dsRNA segments that encode for 13 viral proteins (VP) 1–13. During viral replication, the virus is found in the cell cytoplasm. It is commonly associated with granular structures known as viral VIBs and ordered filaments, tubules, and thread arrays. These viruses are transmitted to vertebrate hosts by tick vectors [35].

4.1.2 Orbiviruses

The Orbivirus genus is the largest within the *Reoviridae* family, comprising 22 species and at least 130 serotypes, which can be differentiated using a virus-neutralization assay. The name "Orbivirus" is derived from the Latin word "Orbis," meaning circle or ring, and reflects the characteristics of this large group of viruses. Orbiviruses can infect a variety of species, including humans, horses, monkeys, rabbits, cattle, deer, and suckling mice. Several types of insects transmit these viruses, including mosquitoes, midges, gnats, sandflies, and ticks, with the BTV being one notable example [40, 41].

Orbivirus disease has been reported infrequently in humans, with fewer than 100 documented cases worldwide. During the maintenance cycle of vector-borne transmission among nonhuman vertebrate hosts, humans can occasionally become incidental hosts for the infection. Various insects, including mosquitoes, midges, gnats, sandflies, and ticks, can transmit the pathogen [40].

The significance of BTV or African horse sickness virus (AHSV) infections in dogs and other carnivores for epidemiological studies is poorly understood. It remains unclear whether these animals develop a significant level of viremia that could be a source of infection for adult Culicoides midges. Serological evidence suggests that AHSV can infect elephants, and positive samples have also been identified in camels, cattle, sheep, and goats. In rare cases, humans have contracted AHSV, leading to conditions such as encephalitis and retinitis, typically resulting from inhaling a freeze-dried neurotropic vaccine strain [42].

BTV, Epizootic hemorrhagic disease virus (EHDV), or AHSV infection typically causes fever and may result in swelling and inflammation, particularly around the face, mouth, and nose. BTV replicates in hematopoietic and lymphoid tissues, including the spleen, bone marrow, monocytes, macrophages, neutrophils, and lymph nodes. Infection of endothelial cells can lead to vascular thrombosis and hemorrhages ranging from petechiae to ecchymosis. Disruption of cell junctions may leak fluid into surrounding tissues or the lungs [43].

CTFV is the virus responsible for Colorado tick fever (CTF), a viral illness primarily found in the western United States and Canada. Approximately 200 to 400 cases are reported each year. CTF is often misdiagnosed and underreported. Currently, there are no approved medications or vaccines; treatment typically involves supportive care and antipyretics. CTF is characterized by biphasic fever, chills, headache, photophobia, and muscle aches, and it may also present with a petechial rash. Due to the severity of their symptoms, around 20% of patients require hospitalization. In pediatric cases, the virus can lead to complications such as aseptic meningitis, meningoencephalitis, or encephalitis, with an estimated 5–15% of children experiencing severe central nervous system or hemorrhagic complications [44]. CTF is characterized by the persistent presence of the virus in the bloodstream due to its ability to replicate within certain types of blood cells. These include erythroblasts, reticulocytes, and CD34+ hematopoietic progenitor cells [45].

5. Immune evasion

BTV is one of the most extensively studied orbiviruses within the *Reoviridae* family. Like other viruses, the replication can be inhibited in vitro by adding endogenous IFN. Treating cells with IFN before BTV infection can also hinder the virus's replication. Both type I IFNs (IFN-I) (alpha and beta) and type II IFN (IFN-II) gamma (Y) can protect cells from viral infections. However, reoviruses have developed strategies to evade the immune response by inhibiting the action of interferons. This means that the virus can still replicate even in the presence of IFN, indicating that it has mechanisms to block the effects of these immune signals [46].

Evidence indicates that the early induction of IFN reduces the replication of BTV in infected calves. However, as serum IFN levels decline, the viral titers tend to increase. Initially, the virulence appears to be suppressed by the action of IFN-I, but it peaks again when the IFN response diminishes. Transcriptome analysis has also shown that the decrease in T cells by day 7 post-infection (7 pi) is associated with the immune activation of the IFN pathway [47].

Studies on cell function indicate that BTV inhibits the proliferation of CD4+ and CD8+ T cells. This finding aligns with the upregulation of programmed cell death ligand 1 (PD-L1) observed on monocytes and CD4+ and CD8+ T cells. These data suggest that BTV may use the PD1/PD-L1 immune checkpoint to inhibit T cells [47, 48].

Other studies have shown that BTV causes acute immunosuppression by infecting and destroying follicular dendritic cells (FDCs) and reducing the capabilities of granulocytes (GCs), which affects antibody production [49].

6. *Asfarviridae*: General features, replication cycle, and immune evasion strategies

The *Asfarviridae* family is the only one that consists of double-stranded deoxyribonucleic acid (dsDNA) viruses. Within this family, ASFV is the sole member of the Asfivirus genus. African swine fever (ASF) is a highly contagious and often lethal disease that affects domestic pigs, warthogs, wild boars, and bush pigs (**Table 1**).

The virus is primarily transmitted through soft ticks of the *Ornithodoros* genus (*Ornithodoros moubata*), as well as through direct contact with infected animals or contaminated surfaces (fomites) and by ingesting contaminated animal by-products. The virus is maintained in wild warthogs and Ornithodoros soft ticks, which serve as natural reservoirs, allowing the infection to persist for an extended period in a sylvatic cycle. The virus can be transmitted in ticks across different life stages (transstadial transmission), between males and females (transovarial transmission), and vertically from parents to offspring. However, transmission from these soft ticks is generally limited to areas near wildlife, as the ticks will feed on their mammalian hosts before dropping off. There is a higher risk of spread and infection when wild boar populations come into close contact with wild pig populations.

Depending on the virus and host response, the disease can manifest from subacute to chronic, resulting in hemorrhagic fever and a fatality rate close to 100% in infected domestic pigs. Pathologies associated with this condition include skin redness, swelling, and bleeding in the lungs, spleen, kidneys, and bladder. Infection is also characterized by thrombocytopenia, destruction of vascular endothelial cells, and the upregulation of apoptosis in infected tissues and blood [50]. This virus is not transmitted to humans.

The virus was first identified in Kenya in the 1920s and remained endemic only in Africa for several decades [51]. However, since the African ASF epidemic began in Georgia in 2007, the virus has spread across Europe, Asia, and parts of the Caribbean. ASF is a notifiable disease to the World Organization for Animal Health (WOAH). By 2020, ASF had been reported in 44 countries, including China, Oceania, Papua New Guinea, the Dominican Republic, and Haiti. The absence of effective treatments or vaccines against the ASF virus has resulted in significant economic losses within the swine industry.

The ASFV is a large, enveloped virus with a dsDNA genome of 170–194 Kb, has approximately 150 ORFs, encodes 150–200 proteins (including 68 SP and over 100 nsP), contains terminal inverted repeats at both ends, and is closed by hairpin loops [52, 53]. ASFV has a complex icosahedral structure, with viral particles measuring approximately 260 nm in size. It features four concentric domains that range from 70 to 100 nm in diameter. The virus is enveloped by a thick layer of protein known as the core-shell, an inner lipid envelope, and an outer icosahedral capsid that forms the exterior of the intracellular virions. ASFV has a genome structure and replication process similar to other large dsDNA viruses, including the *Poxviridae*, *Iridoviridae*, and *Phycodnaviridae* families [50]. One relevant protein associated with the virus particle is the attachment protein p12, which is localized in the outer envelope [54]; the protein p72, a major component of capsomers [55]; and the structural membrane protein pB428L, localized in the capsid [56]. The membrane proteins p54, p17, pE248R, and p12 are found in the inner envelope, with p12 linked to viral membrane precursors, particle assembly, and the formation of intracellular mature viruses. The core-shell processes products from polyproteins pp220 and pp62, while the nucleoid contains DNA-binding proteins p10 and pA104R and the transcriptional machinery required for RNA synthesis and modification.

ASFV replicates in the cytoplasmic viral assembly sites near the porcine monocyte nucleus-macrophage cells. However, there is evidence that viral DNA synthesis can also occur in the nucleus during the early stages of infection [57, 58]. The virus enters macrophages and monocytes through various types of endocytosis, including clathrin-mediated dynamin-dependent endocytosis, phagocytosis, and micropinocytosis, which triggers the infection cycle [59]. To achieve endosomal maturation, proteins and lipids are recruited to the endosomal membrane, where capsid disassembly occurs at the acidic pH of the endosomal lumen [60]. The core particle includes RNA polymerase, which is essential for early gene transcription required for virus replication and the suppression of host defense mechanisms. Moreover, the ubiquitin-proteasome system plays a role in the degradation of the final capsid, allowing the viral DNA to be released into the host cytoplasm, where

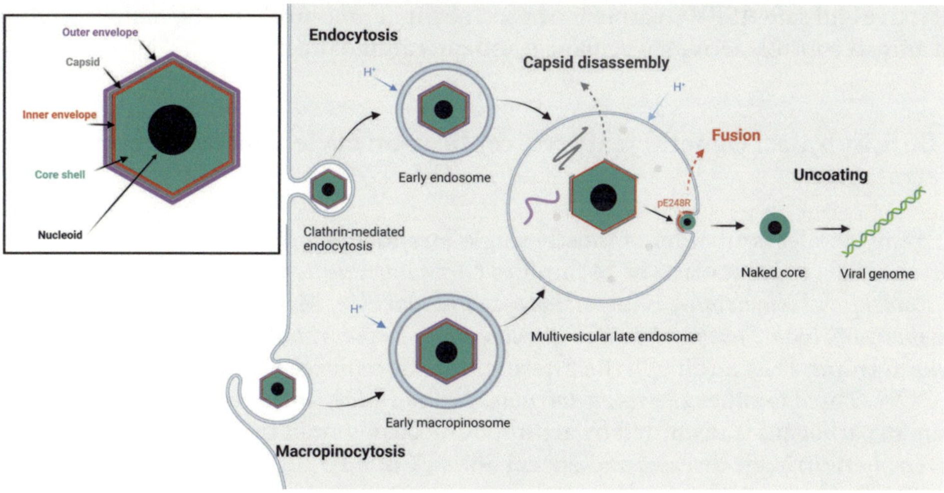

Figure 4.
Schematic representation of the replication cycle of Asfarviridae. *ASFV enters macrophages and monocytes through clathrin-mediated, dynamin-dependent endocytosis and actin-driven micropinocytosis. Following entry, the virus goes through a process of unwrapping via the endocytic pathway. To achieve endosomal maturation, proteins and lipids are recruited to the endosomal membrane, and capsid disassembly occurs at the acidic pH of the endosomal lumen. The disassembly process involves the dissociation of the outer envelope (purple), disruption of the capsid (gray), and fusion of the inner viral envelope (red). The membrane protein pE248R mediates membrane fusion and core delivery. After fusion, the naked core is delivered into the cytosol to continue the uncoating process until the viral genome is released.*

replication begins (**Figure 4**) [61]. The mature particle travels to the cell surface through a microtubule-mediated mechanism, and then it is released to the host cell by budding at the cell membrane.

6.1 Immune evasion

ASFV primarily targets macrophages and monocytes, which limits the range of cells it can infect. These cell types present antigens to T cells, triggering innate immune responses and activating the adaptive immune response. ASFV encodes enzymes in the DNA base excision repair (BER) pathway to bypass the replication barriers found in macrophages [62]. ASFV has multiple IFN-I and IFN-II inhibitor genes necessary to recognize pathogen-associated molecular patterns (PAMPs) [63]. The inhibition of IFN compromises the activation of the JAK-STAT pathway, which restricts virus replication through innate and adaptive responses [64]. The ER plays a vital role in replicating ASFV. When proteins accumulate in this compartment, it causes stress and triggers the unfolded protein response (UPR) in host cells, which aims to limit viral replication. To counteract this response, ASFV promotes the upregulation of chaperones, specifically calnexin and calreticulin, to enhance the folding capacity of the ER. ASFV modulates apoptosis, a critical host response to limit replication and viral spread by inducing cell death. The ASFV gene encodes Bcl-2, an anti-apoptotic protein inhibiting apoptosis [65] and autophagy by interacting with Beclin 1 through BH3 homolog.

Understanding how the virus interacts with and modifies the host response during infection is crucial for developing novel vaccines. Various approaches have been attempted to create an effective ASFV vaccine, including inactivated, live attenuated, genetically engineered subunit, DNA, and vector vaccines. The absence of an effective and safe ASFV treatment or vaccine hinders control efforts, mainly relying on animal control, active surveillance, and quarantine practices.

7. Bunyavirales: General features, replication cycle, and immune evasion strategies

Bunyavirales is an order of mostly single-stranded, tri-segmented RNA viruses. This order consists of 14 families (*Arenaviridae, Cruliviridae, Discoviridae, Fimoviridae, Hantaviridae, Leishbuviridae, Mypoviridae, Nairoviridae, Peribunyaviridae, Phasmaviridae, Phenuiviridae, Tospoviridae, Tulsaviridae, and Wupedieviridae*) according to the International Committee on Taxonomy of Viruses (ICTV). Three families (*Peribunyaviridae, Nairoviridae,* and *Phenuiviridae*) contain human pathogens transmitted by arthropods, causing mild to severe diseases such as fevers, hemorrhagic disease, and encephalitis (**Table 1**) [66].

The *Peribunyaviridae* family has four genera: *Orthobunyavirus*, *Herbesvirus*, *Pacuvirus*, and *Shangavirus*. The *Orthobunyavirus* genus is the most studied and understood of the family. It includes viruses such as California encephalitis virus (CEV), La Crosse encephalitis virus (LACV), Bunyamwera virus (BUNV), Ngari virus (NRIV), Batai virus (BATV), and Oropouche virus (OROV). The viruses can cause various human symptoms, from mild fever to encephalitis. In ruminants, they may result in abortions. These viruses are now considered a growing global health concern due to the changing environmental conditions caused by climate change, which supports the spread of vectors [67].

One virus that has recently been shown to be of great interest and importance in terms of its impact on public health is the OROV. This virus is spread by arthropod vectors and is mainly found in the tropical regions of Central and South America. During an outbreak, the virus was first detected in 1955 near the Oropuche River in Trinidad and Tobago. Since then, it has led to epidemics in South and Central America, impacting countries such as Brazil, Bolivia, Panama, Peru, Ecuador, French Guiana, and, most recently, Cuba. Between January and July of 2024, a total of 7700 confirmed cases of this virus have been reported, with the majority occurring in Brazil, followed by Bolivia, Peru, Cuba, and Colombia [68].

OROV is transmitted to humans by the bite of an infected female mosquito from Culicoides. It is believed that OROV has a sylvatic replication cycle involving primates, sloths, and possibly some bird species. However, the primary mosquito vector has not yet been identified. In the human infection cycle, OROV is primarily transmitted by *Culicoides paraensis*, with *Culex quinquefasciatus* serving as a secondary vector [68, 69].

A couple of studies indicate that symptoms can reoccur in approximately 60% of patients who have recovered from OROV infection, typically 1 or 2 weeks later. Furthermore, this infection may lead to specific hemorrhagic symptoms and neurological complications. One area still being studied is vertical transmission in humans. There have been reported cases of abortions and fetal deaths associated with OROV infection [70].

Currently, no specific treatment or vaccine is available for this viral infection. The most effective approach is to manage the symptoms and provide supportive care.

The *Nairoviridae* family includes known human pathogens such as the Crimean-Congo Hemorrhagic Fever virus (CCHFV) and nonhuman pathogenic viruses, including the Dugbe virus (DUGV), Nairobi Sheep Disease virus (NSDV), and Hazara virus (HAZV). These viruses have similarities in how they are transmitted in the environment and how their genetic material is organized. Ticks maintain and transmit hosts, including birds, humans, rodents, and ruminants. *Nairoviridae*, compared to other bunyaviruses, have a more complex genome. They are closely related to the Bunyavirales family. Only one virus in this family was identified in July 2019: Wuhan millipede virus 2 [71].

The *Phenuiviridae* family includes animals, plants, insects, and human pathogens. Generally, viruses are transmitted by ticks or sandflies. However, the RVFV is an exception and is transmitted by mosquitoes. RVFV can cause mild to severe symptoms in humans and animals, such as febrile illness, meningitis, hemorrhagic fever, hepatitis, hemorrhage, and abortion in cattle and sheep [72].

The *Bunyaviridae* family consists of icosahedral, enveloped viruses that measure 100–120 nm in diameter. They possess tripartite negative-sense single-stranded RNA (-ssRNA) genomes of negative sense, which are referred to as the large (L), medium (M), and small (S) segments. The L RNA contains the RdRp present in the virion. The L protein of the Crimean-Congo hemorrhagic fever virus encodes an ovarian tumor-like cysteine protease motif, suggesting that the L polyprotein is cleaved autoproteolytically. The mRNA encodes two glycoproteins, light cyan glycoprotein (Gc) and dark cyan glycoprotein (Gn), found on the surface of virions. The sRNA encodes a nucleocapsid protein [73].

All stages of viral replication occur in the cytoplasm. The replication cycle begins with viral attachment to the host receptor, mediated by an interaction of

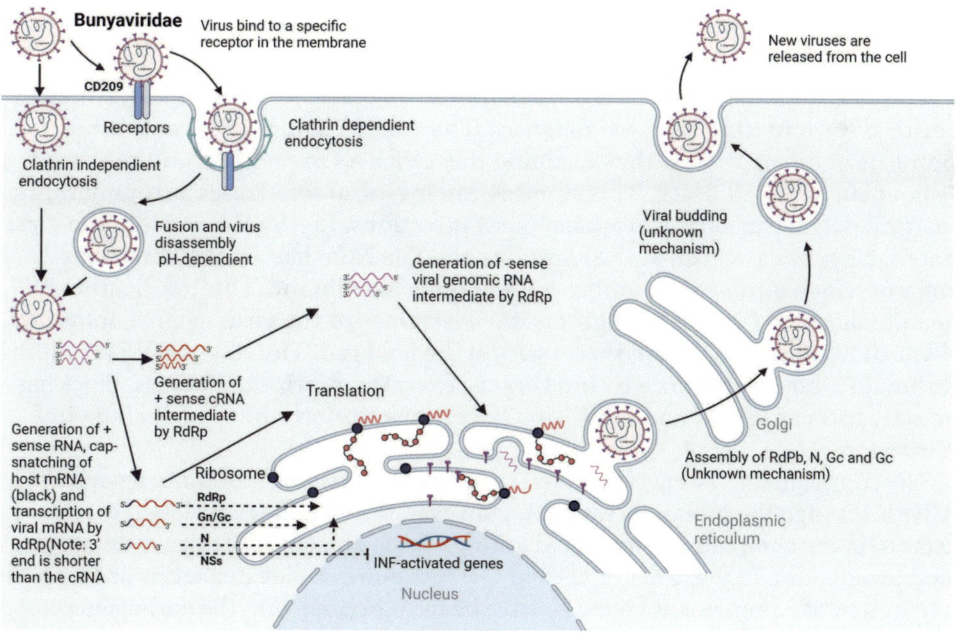

Figure 5.
Schematic representation of the replication cycle of Bunyaviridae. *Bunyavirus infects a cell through receptor-mediated endocytosis, which may involve clathrin or clathrin-independent endocytosis. Upon viral entry, uncoating of the virion results in the presentation of multisegmented (−) sense RNA in the host cytoplasm. The RdRp in the viral particle facilitates replication of the genome into a positive-sense RNA intermediate. The process of "cap-snatching" allows 5′ host mRNA to attach and create viral mRNA that can be translated. The mRNA creates all the necessary parts for an infectious virus, including glycoproteins N, C, nucleoprotein, and RdRp. It can also create up to two NS proteins, NSs and NSm. The (+) sense intermediate RNA can also serve as a template for genomic replication by the RdRp into (−) sense genomic RNA.*

one or both integral viral envelope proteins, which remain unidentified (**Figure 5**). The next step involves the entry and uncoating of virions through endocytosis, followed by the fusion of viral membranes with endosomal membranes. The RdRp synthesizes new mRNA to be used as complementary genome templates, utilizing capped primers obtained from the host cell. The translation of primary L and S segment mRNAs by free ribosomes, translation of M segment mRNAs by membrane-bound ribosomes, and primary glycosylation of nascent envelope proteins result in the synthesis of all the components of an infectious virus (i.e., glycoprotein N, glycoprotein C, nucleoprotein, and RdRp) as well as up to two NS proteins, nonstructural S segment (NSs) and nonstructural M segment protein (NSm). The viral RNA serves as a matrix for both replication and transcription processes. Positive-sense RNA replicative intermediates are utilized to produce more copies for progeny. Replicative intermediates are full-length template strands that have 6–8 daughter strands emerging from them. The morphogenesis process involves accumulating Gn and Gc in the Golgi, terminal glycosylation, and acquiring modified host membranes. This process often occurs through budding into the Golgi cisternae. The ribonucleoproteins of tomato spotted wilt virus (genus Tospovirus) are surrounded by complete stacks of the Golgi apparatus. This leads to the formation of virus particles that are doubly enveloped. These particles subsequently fuse with the ER to create large vesicles derived from this compartment. These vesicles contain substantial quantities of mature, singly enveloped tospovirus particles (**Figure 5**) [74, 75].

7.1 Immune evasion

The LACV, CCHFV, and RVFV can suppress the production of IFN-I, which is critical for initiating antiviral defenses. The CCHFV and RVFV can inhibit apoptosis in infected cells, thus enabling these viruses to replicate and propagate without eliciting cell death. This suppression is crucial for viruses as it undermines a natural defense mechanism against viral infections. In RVFV infection, the viral protein NSm has a crucial anti-apoptotic role. The NSm has a transmembrane domain, which binds to the mitochondrial outer membrane. This localization to the mitochondria further strengthens the resistance of the virus against apoptosis, which allows it to persist and thrive within the host cell. The NSs of RVFV suppress the innate immune response by binding to several transcription factors, blocking the activation of IFN-β, and inhibiting host transcription while improving viral translation [72].

The complement system is essential in offering protective immunity against CCHFV through the humoral response. However, the virus has developed mechanisms to evade complement-mediated killing. These evasion strategies result in a notable reduction in the levels of C3 and C4. Intriguingly, elevated levels of factor Bb (a fragment of complement factor B) have been associated with the pathogenesis of the disease [76].

T cell responses in patients infected with *Phenuiviridae* viruses have shown that non-survivors exhibit decreased T cell counts, indicating immune dysfunction, while survivors display heightened activation markers and stronger antiviral responses. Research on the CCHFV has identified CD4+ and CD8+ T cell-specific epitopes within the CCHFV glycoprotein precursor (GPC), nucleoprotein (N), and RdRp. Notably, strong IFN-γ responses against the NSm region of the GP38 protein have been observed in CCHFV survivors, indicating immune activation [77].

8. Remarks and conclusions

Vector-borne diseases (VBD) are human and animal illnesses caused by viruses, parasites, and bacteria transmitted by vectors. A vector is a living organism capable of transmitting infectious pathogens. The arboviruses are the leading cause of VBD public health burden globally. They include a wide range of virus families and subfamilies. One important characteristic is that blood-sucking insects like mosquitoes and ticks can transmit them. These viruses can infect, replicate, and evade the immune system in mammals and invertebrates, thus continuing the infection cycle [1]. The dramatic increase in the emergence and reemergence of arboviruses has created a global public health emergency, costing the lives of millions of people and threatening economic security globally [78].

The study of arbovirus replication cycles helps us understand how these viruses control the host cell machinery and avoid the immune system. Although we have some understanding of their processes, there are still aspects of each disease that remain unclear. Uncovering the molecular mechanisms involved and the biological interaction between arboviruses and host immune response can provide significant knowledge for developing effective vaccines and treatments and implementing control and prevention approaches against arboviruses [79, 80]. Although there is much to continue discovering, there is no doubt that the study of these entities is exciting.

Acknowledgements

The authors come from various academic and research institutions. Each author expresses gratitude for the financial support, knowledge, and professional preparation provided by their respective institutions.

Conflict of interest

The authors declare no conflict of interest.

Acronyms

+dsRNA	positive-sense double-stranded RNA
+ssRNA	positive-sense single-stranded RNA
-ssRNA	negative-sense single-stranded RNA
Arboviruses	arthropod-borne viruses
AHSV	African horse sickness virus
ASF	African swine fever
ASFV	African swine fever virus
ASP3	aspartyl protease 3
AUD	alphavirus unique domain
BATV	Batai virus
BER	base excision repair
BUNV	Bunyamwera virus
C	capsid
CCHFV	Crimean-Congo hemorrhagic fever virus

CEV	California encephalitis virus
CHIKV	Chikungunya virus
CTF	Colorado trick fever
CTFV	Colorado trick fever virus
DENV	dengue virus
DICAM	dual Ig domain-containing cell adhesion molecule
DNA	deoxyribonucleic acid
dsRNA	double-stranded RNA
dsDNA	Double-stranded DNA
DUGV	Dugbe virus
E	envelope protein
EHDV	epizootic hemorrhagic disease virus
EIP	extrinsic incubation period
ER	endoplasmic reticulum
FDC	follicular dendritic cell
GCs	granulocytes
Gc	light cyan glycoprotein
Gn	dark cyan glycoprotein
GPC	glycoprotein precursor
HAZV	Hazara virus
ICTV	International Committee on Taxonomy of Viruses
IFN	interferon
IL	interleukins
IMD	immune deficiency pathway
JAK-STAT	Janus Kinase-signal transducer and activator of transcription
VIBs	viral inclusion bodies
JEV	Japanese encephalitis virus
LACV	La Crosse encephalitis virus
MAYV	Mayaro virus
MCP-1	Monocyte chemoattractant protein-1
Mxra8	matrix remodeling associate 8
NOS	reactive nitrogen species
NRIV	Ngari virus
NS	nonstructural
NSDV	Nairobi sheep disease virus
nsP	nonstructural protein
NSm	nonstructural M segment protein
NSs	nonstructural S segment protein
OROV	oropouche virus
ORF	open reading frame
PD-L1	programmed cell death ligand 1
pRM	precursor membrane
PO	phenoloxidase
RC	replication complex
RdRp	RNA-dependent RNA polymerase
RIG-1	retinoic acid-inducible gene 1
RNA	ribonucleic acid
RNAi	RNA interference
ROS	reactive oxygen species
RVFV	rift valley fever virus

SINV	Sindbis virus
ssRNA	single-stranded RNA
SP	structural proteins
STING	stimulator of interferon genes
TEPs	thioester-containing proteins
TF	transframe protein
TLR3	toll-like receptor 3
UPR	unfolded protein response
UTR	untranslated regions
VP	viral proteins
WEEV	Western equine encephalitis virus
WNV	West Nile virus
YFV	yellow fever virus
ZIKV	Zika virus

Author details

Manuel Alejandro Mosso Pani[1], Henry Puerta-Guardo[2], Daniel Nunez-Avellaneda[3], Nicole M. Nazario Maldonado[4] and Luis Antonio Alonso-Palomares[4]*

1 Laboratory of Genomics, ODIN Bioscience, Miami, Florida, United States of America

2 Virology Lab, Centro de Investigaciones Regionales "Dr. Hideyo Noguchi", Universidad Autonoma de Yucatan (UADY), Mérida, Yucatán, México

3 Deputy General Direction for Technological Development, Cooperation and Innovation, National Council of Humanities, Sciences and Technologies, Mexico City, Mexico

4 Infectious Diseases and Immunology Department, College of Veterinary Medicine, University of Florida, Gainesville, Florida, United States of America

*Address all correspondence to: luis_alp88@hotmail.com

References

[1] Chala B, Hamde F. Emerging and re-emerging vector-borne infectious diseases and the challenges for control: A review. Frontiers in Public Health. 2021;**9**. DOI: 10.3389/fpubh.2021.715759

[2] Viglietta M, Bellone R, Blisnick AA, Failloux AB. Vector specificity of arbovirus transmission. Frontiers in Microbiology. 2021;**12**. DOI: 10.3389/fmicb.2021.773211

[3] Sick F, Beer M, Kampen H, Wernike K. Culicoides biting midges—Underestimated vectors for arboviruses of public health and veterinary importance. Viruses. 2019;**11**. DOI: 10.3390/v11040376

[4] Alonso-Palomares LA, Moreno-García M, Lanz-Mendoza H, Salazar MI. Molecular basis for arbovirus transmission by *Aedes aegypti* mosquitoes. Intervirology. 2019;**61**:255-264. DOI: 10.1159/000499128

[5] Wu P, Yu X, Wang P, Cheng G. Arbovirus lifecycle in mosquito: Acquisition, propagation and transmission. Expert Reviews in Molecular Medicine. 2019;**21**. DOI: 10.1017/erm.2018.6

[6] Neufeldt CJ, Cortese M, Acosta EG, Bartenschlager R. Rewiring cellular networks by members of the *Flaviviridae* family. Nature Reviews Microbiology. 2018;**16**. DOI: 10.1038/nrmicro.2017.170

[7] Kalia M, Khasa R, Sharma M, Nain M, Vrati S. Japanese encephalitis virus infects neuronal cells through a clathrin-independent endocytic mechanism. Journal of Virology. 2013;**87**:148-162

[8] Yu Y, Si L, Meng Y. Flavivirus entry inhibitors. Advances in Experimental Medicine and Biology. 2022;**1366**:171-197

[9] Wang QY, Shi PY. Flavivirus entry inhibitors. ACS Infectious Diseases. 2016;**1**:428-434

[10] Aviner R, Li KH, Frydman J, Andino R. Cotranslational prolyl hydroxylation is essential for flavivirus biogenesis. Nature. 2021;**596**:558-564

[11] Chen S et al. Flaviviridae virus nonstructural proteins 5 and 5A mediate viral immune evasion and are promising targets in drug development. Pharmacology and Therapeutics. 2018;**190**:1-14. DOI: 10.1016/j.pharmthera.2018.05.004

[12] Wu J, Liu W, Gong P, Gong P. A structural overview of RNA-dependent RNA polymerases from the *Flaviviridae* family. International Journal of Molecular Sciences. 2015;**16**:12943-12957. DOI: 10.3390/ijms160612943

[13] Zhang Q-Y et al. Short direct repeats in the 3′ untranslated region are involved in subgenomic flaviviral RNA production. Journal of Virology. 2020;**94**

[14] Uchil PD, Kumar AVA, Satchidanandam V. Nuclear localization of flavivirus RNA synthesis in infected cells. Journal of Virology. 2006;**80**:5451-5464

[15] De Jesús-González LA et al. Nucleo-cytoplasmic transport of ZIKV non-structural 3 protein is mediated by importin-α/β and exportin CRM-1. Journal of Virology. 2023;**97**

[16] Reyes-Ruiz JM et al. Strand-like structures and the nonstructural proteins 5, 3 and 1 are present in the nucleus of mosquito cells infected with dengue virus. Virology. 2018;**515**:74-80

[17] Bhuvanakantham R, Cheong YK, Ng ML. West Nile virus capsid protein interaction with importin and HDM2 protein is regulated by protein kinase C-mediated phosphorylation. Microbes and Infection. 2010;**12**:615-625

[18] De Jesús-González LA et al. The nuclear pore complex is a key target of viral proteases to promote viral replication. Viruses. 2021;**13**. DOI: 10.3390/v13040706

[19] Paul D, Bartenschlager R. *Flaviviridae* replication organelles: Oh, what a tangled web we weave. Annual Review of Virology. 2015;**2**. DOI: 10.1146/annurev-virology-100114-055007

[20] Mukhopadhyay S, Kuhn RJ, Rossmann MG. A structural perspective of the flavivirus life cycle. Nature Reviews Microbiology. 2005;**3**:289-310. DOI: 10.1038/nrmicro1067

[21] Neufeldt CJ et al. ER-shaping atlastin proteins act as central hubs to promote flavivirus replication and virion assembly. Nature Microbiology. 2019;**4**:13-22

[22] Diosa-Toro M, Prasanth KR, Bradrick SS, Garcia Blanco MA. Role of RNA-binding proteins during the late stages of flavivirus replication cycle. Virology Journal. 2020;**17**

[23] Kanojia A, Sharma M, Shiraz R, Tripathi S. Flavivirus–host interaction landscape visualized through genome-wide CRISPR screens. Viruses. 2022;**14**:2416-2429. DOI: 10.3390/v14102164

[24] Uno N, Ross TM. Dengue virus and the host innate immune response. Emerging Microbes and Infections. 2018;**7**. DOI: 10.1038/s41426-018-0168-0

[25] dos Peinado RS, Eberle RJ, Arni RK, Coronado MA. A review of omics studies on arboviruses: alphavirus, orthobunyavirus and phlebovirus. Viruses. 2022;**14**. DOI: 10.3390/v14102194

[26] Pietilä MK, Hellström K, Ahola T. Alphavirus polymerase and RNA replication. Virus Research. 2017;**234**:44-57

[27] Holmes AC, Basore K, Fremont DH, Diamond MS. A molecular understanding of alphavirus entry. PLoS Pathogens. 2020;**16**:1-20

[28] Zhang R et al. Mxra8 is a receptor for multiple arthritogenic alphaviruses. Nature. 2018;**557**

[29] Mendes A, Kuhn RJ. Alphavirus nucleocapsid packaging and assembly. Viruses. 2018;**10**:1-15

[30] Fortuna C et al. Vector competence of *Aedes albopictus* for the Indian Ocean lineage (IOL) chikungunya viruses of the 2007 and 2017 outbreaks in Italy: A comparison between strains with and without the E1: A226V mutation. Eurosurveillance. 2018;**23**

[31] Baxter VK, Heise MT. Immunopathogenesis of alphaviruses. Advances in Virus Research (United States, Germany, United Kingdom). 2020;**107**:315-382. DOI: 10.1016/bs.aivir.2020.06.002. Epub 2020 Jul 8

[32] Joklik WK. The members of the family *Reoviridae*. In: Joklik WK, editor. The Reoviridae. The Viruses (VIRS Series). Boston, MA: Springer; 1983. pp. 1-7. DOI: 10.1007/978-1-4899-0580-2_1

[33] Matsuo E, Roy P. Minimum requirements for bluetongue virus primary replication *in vivo*. Journal of Virology. 2013;**87**:1-14

[34] Stuart DI, Grimes JM. Structural studies on orbivirus proteins and particles. Current Topics in Microbiology and Immunology. 2006;**309**:3961-3972. DOI: 10.1007/3-540-30773-7_8

[35] Attoui H, Jaafar FM, De Micco P, De Lamballerie X. Coltiviruses and Seadornaviruses in North America, Europe, and Asia. Emerging Infectious Diseases. 2005;**11**:179-196. DOI: 10.3201/eid1111.050868

[36] Yadav PD et al. Characterization of novel Reoviruses wad Medani virus (Orbivirus) and Kundal virus (Coltivirus) collected from Hyalomma anatolicum ticks in India during surveillance for Crimean Congo hemorrhagic fever. Journal of Virology. 2019;**93**:1673-1679

[37] Weiss S, Dabrowski PW, Kurth A, Leendertz SAJ, Leendertz FH. A novel coltivirus-related virus isolated from free-tailed bats from Côte d'Ivoire is able to infect human cells in vitro. Virology Journal. 2017;**14**

[38] Fujita R et al. Isolation and characterization of Tarumizu tick virus: A new coltivirus from Haemaphysalis flava ticks in Japan. Virus Research. 2017;**242**

[39] Schoch CL et al. NCBI taxonomy: A comprehensive update on curation, resources and tools. Database. 2020;**2020**. DOI: 10.1093/database/baaa062

[40] DeBiasi RL, Tyler KL. Orthoreoviruses and orbiviruses. In: Mandell, Douglas, and Bennett's Principles and Practice of Infectious Diseases. Amsterdam, Netherlands: Elsevier; 2015. pp. 1848-1850.e1. DOI: 10.1016/B978-1-4557-4801-3.00150-8. Epub 2014 Oct 31

[41] Wilson AJ, Mellor PS. Bluetongue in Europe: Past, present and future. Philosophical Transactions of the Royal Society B: Biological Sciences. 2009;**364**:1835-1842. DOI: 10.1098/rstb.2009.0091

[42] Barnard BJ, Bengis RG, Keet DF, Dekker EH. Epidemiology of African horsesickness: Antibodies in free-living elephants (*Loxodonta africans*) and their response to experimental infection. The Onderstepoort Journal of Veterinary Research. 1995;**62**:2669-2681

[43] Zientara S, Weyer CT, Lecollinet S. African horse sickness. OIE Revue Scientifique et Technique. 2015;**34**:37-42

[44] Brackney MM et al. Epidemiology of Colorado tick fever in Montana, Utah, and Wyoming, 1995-2003. Vector-Borne and Zoonotic Diseases. 2010;**10**:569-581

[45] Owen S et al. Colorado tick fever virus induces apoptosis in human endothelial cells to facilitate viral replication. Ticks and Tick-Borne Diseases. 2021;**12**:291-296

[46] Vitour D et al. Induction and control of the type I interferon pathway by Bluetongue virus. Virus Research. 2014;**182**:59-70

[47] Smith DR, Jones AT, Long J, et al. Innate immune responses of calves during transient infection with bovine viral diarrhea virus. Veterinary Research. 2012;**43**:19. DOI: 10.1186/1297-9716-43-19

[48] Melzi E et al. Follicular dendritic cell disruption as a novel mechanism

of virus-induced immunosuppression. Proceedings of the National Academy of Sciences of the United States of America. 2016;**113**:E6238-E6247

[49] Louloudes-Lázaro A et al. Comprehensive immune profiling reveals that orbivirus infection activates immune checkpoints during acute T cell immunosuppression. Frontiers in Immunology. 2023;**14**:E6238-E6247

[50] Dixon LK, Sun H, Roberts H. African swine fever. Antiviral Research. 2019;**165**. DOI: 10.1016/j.antiviral.2019.02.018

[51] Eustace Montgomery R. On a form of swine fever occurring in British East Africa (Kenya Colony). Journal of Comparative Pathology and Therapeutics. 1921;**34**:34-41

[52] Alejo A, Matamoros T, Guerra M, Andrés G. A proteomic atlas of the African swine fever virus particle. Journal of Virology. 2018;**92**:159-191

[53] Chapman DAG et al. Genomic analysis of highly virulent Georgia 2007/1 isolate of African swine fever virus. Emerging Infectious Diseases. 2011;**17**

[54] Carrascosa AL, Saastre I, González P, Viñuela E. Localization of the African swine fever virus attachment protein p12 in the virus particle by immunoelectron microscopy. Virology. 1993;**193**:599-605

[55] García-Escudero R, Andrés G, Almazán F, Viñuela E. Inducible gene expression from African swine fever virus recombinants: Analysis of the major capsid protein p72. Journal of Virology. 1998;**72**:615-624

[56] Epifano C, Krijnse-Locker J, Salas ML, Salas J, Rodríguez JM. Generation of filamentous instead of icosahedral particles by repression of African swine fever virus structural protein pB438L. Journal of Virology. 2006;**80**:8988-8994

[57] García-Beato R, Salas ML, Viñuela E, Salas J. Role of the host cell nucleus in the replication of African swine fever virus DNA. Virology. 1992;**188**:12260-12267

[58] Rojo G, García-Beato R, Viñuela E, Salas ML, Salas J. Replication of African swine fever virus DNA in infected cells. Virology. 1999;**257**:646-655

[59] Galindo I et al. African swine fever virus infects macrophages, the natural host cells, via clathrin- and cholesterol-dependent endocytosis. Virus Research. 2015;**200**:414-425

[60] Cuesta-Geijo MA et al. Endosomal maturation, Rab7 GTPase and phosphoinositides in African swine fever virus entry. PLoS One. 2012;**7**:45-55

[61] Barrado-Gil L, Galindo I, Martínez-Alonso D, Viedma S, Alonso C. The ubiquitin-proteasome system is required for African swine fever replication. PLoS One. 2017;**12**

[62] Dixon LK, Chapman DAG, Netherton CL, Upton C. African swine fever virus replication and genomics. Virus Research. 2013;**173**. DOI: 10.1016/j.virusres.2012.10.020

[63] Correia S, Ventura S, Parkhouse RM. Identification and utility of innate immune system evasion mechanisms of ASFV. Virus Research. 2013;**173**:3-14. DOI: 10.1016/j.virusres.2012.10.013

[64] Randall RE, Goodbourn S. Interferons and viruses: An interplay between induction, signalling, antiviral responses and virus countermeasures. Journal of General Virology. 2008;**89**:87-100. DOI: 10.1099/vir.0.83391-0

[65] Brun A, Rivas C, Esteban M, Escribano JM, Alonso C. African swine fever virus gene A179L, a viral homologue of bcl-2, protects cells from programmed cell death. Virology. 1996;**225**:1-47

[66] Abudurexiti A et al. Taxonomy of the order Bunyavirales: Update 2019. Archives of Virology. 2019;**164**:227-237

[67] Hughes HR et al. ICTV virus taxonomy profile: *Peribunyaviridae*. Journal of General Virology. 2020;**101**:1949-1965

[68] Romero-Alvarez D, Escobar LE. Oropouche fever, an emergent disease from the Americas. Microbes and Infection. 2018;**20**:779-780. DOI: 10.1016/j.micinf.2017.11.013

[69] Romero-Alvarez D, Escobar LE, Auguste AJ, Del Valle SY, Manore CA. Transmission risk of Oropouche fever across the Americas. Infectious Diseases of Poverty. 2023;**12**:135-146

[70] Tilston-Lunel NL. Oropouche virus: An emerging Orthobunyavirus. The Journal of General Virology. 2024;**105**. DOI: 10.1099/jgv.0.002027

[71] Garrison AR et al. ICTV virus taxonomy profile: *Nairoviridae*. Journal of General Virology. 2020;**101**

[72] Rima B et al. ICTV virus taxonomy profile: *Pneumoviridae*. Journal of General Virology. 2017;**98**:798-799

[73] Leventhal SS, Wilson D, Feldmann H, Hawman DW. A look into bunyavirales genomes: Functions of non-structural (ns) proteins. Viruses. 2021;**13**:291-292. DOI: 10.3390/v13020314

[74] Boshra H. An overview of the infectious cycle of bunyaviruses. Viruses. 2022;**14**. DOI: 10.3390/v14102139

[75] Horne KME, Vanlandingham DL. Bunyavirus-vector interactions. Viruses. 2014;**6**. DOI: 10.3390/v6114373

[76] Rodriguez SE et al. Immunobiology of Crimean-Congo hemorrhagic fever. Antiviral Research. 2022;**199**:4373-4390. DOI: 10.1016/j.antiviral.2022.105244

[77] Alatrash R, Herrera BB. The adaptive immune response against bunyavirales. Viruses. 2024;**16**. DOI: 10.3390/v16030483

[78] Young PR. Arboviruses: A family on the move. Advances in Experimental Medicine and Biology. 2018;**1062**

[79] Lundstrom K. Alphavirus-based vaccines. Viruses. 2014;**6**:2392-2415

[80] Torres-Flores JM, Reyes-Sandoval A, Salazar MI. Dengue vaccines: An update. BioDrugs. 2022;**36**

Section 2

Clinical Aspects, Diagnostics and Miscellaneous

Chapter 4

Giardia intestinalis and Giardiasis: Biological, Immunological and Therapeutic Perspectives

Haleema H. Albohiri, Eman S. Elwakil, Sarah Albalawi and Muslimah N. Alsulami

Abstract

One of the important organisms that significantly contributes to the worldwide disease burden is intestinal parasites, which pose a significant global health issue, affecting at least 20% of the world's population. One of the intestinal parasites that is most prevalent is *Giardia intestinalis*, a flagellated intestinal protozoon, that affects humans, numerous birds, and domestic and wild mammals worldwide. It is also typical in ruminants, such as pigs, dogs, and cats. Giardiasis is ubiquitous in both high-middle-income and low-income nations. It is considered a parasitic disease of enormous epidemiological and clinical importance that causes significant health and economic burdens worldwide. A complicated interaction between innate and adaptive immunological components occurs during the immune response to *G. intestinalis* infection. Correct diagnosis of giardiasis is crucial for effective treatment and prevention of the disease; however, diagnosing *Giardia* infections is challenging because the clinical symptoms are not specific to the illness. As no vaccines are currently available to treat giardiasis, the only treatment available for these infections is chemotherapy with nitroimidazole derivatives including metronidazole, which is the drug used. Although metronidazole treatment is crucial in controlling giardiasis, recent reports have shown the possible formation of resistance to the drug. Medicinal herbs also provide an alternative option for managing *Giardia* infections, as they can offer an efficient treatment with minimal adverse effects compared to other medications.

Keywords: *Giardia intestinalis*, giardiasis, immunology, emerging therapies, drug resistance, diagnostic techniques

1. Introduction

Over the past three decades, infectious diseases have garnered increasing attention from global health organizations such as the World Health Organization (WHO) and the US Institute of Medicine [1]. Various factors have contributed to their growing prevalence, including environmental changes and population growth, which have created favorable conditions for pathogens and increased host-pathogen interactions [2]. These issues are particularly pronounced in low- and middle-income countries (LMICs), where neglected infectious diseases (NIDs) impose a significant burden on public health [3]. Intestinal parasitic infections, a subset of NIDs, affect approximately 20% of the global population and contribute significantly to mortality in developing regions [4, 5].

Among intestinal parasites, *Giardia* is one of the most prevalent and clinically significant. First described by van Leeuwenhoek in 1681, *Giardia* causes giardiasis, a common parasitic disease affecting humans and animals, including ruminants, pigs, and pets [6, 7]. Giardiasis is widespread in LMICs, affecting up to 33% of individuals compared to 2% of adults and 8% of children in industrialized nations [8]. The disease presents significant health and economic challenges, necessitating effective management and prevention strategies [8, 9].

Giardia exhibits a simple life cycle comprising two stages: the infectious cyst and the multiplying trophozoite. Transmission occurs *via* contaminated food, water, or direct fecal-oral contact [10]. Ingested cysts excyst in the host's gastrointestinal tract, releasing trophozoites that colonize the duodenum and jejunum, adhere to the intestinal lining, and multiply, leading to malabsorption and clinical symptoms such as diarrhea, abdominal pain, and weight loss [7, 11]. Severe cases can result in stunted growth, cognitive delays in children, and post-infectious complications like irritable bowel syndrome (IBS) [12]. Globally, *Giardia* ranks as the third leading cause of diarrheal illness, with over 300 million cases annually [13].

Accurate diagnosis is crucial for effective treatment and prevention. Common diagnostic methods include fecal microscopy, immunodiagnostics, and molecular techniques [14]. Standard treatments involve FDA-approved drugs such as metronidazole, tinidazole, and albendazole [15]. However, concerns about drug resistance have sparked interest in alternative therapies, including medicinal herbs, which offer effective treatment with fewer side effects [9].

2. Intestinal parasites

Intestinal parasites (IPIs) are a significant global health challenge, impacting millions of people across various regions and socioeconomic groups [16]. Despite progress in diagnostic techniques, IPIs remain a burden on healthcare systems worldwide [17]. Approximately 3.5 billion individuals are infected, leading to over 450 million cases of illness annually [18]. IPIs primarily consist of helminths and protozoa, residing in the digestive tracts of humans and animals. They are transmitted through the fecal-oral route, often *via* contaminated food or water [18, 19].

Protozoan parasites, comprising about 10,000 species, include common pathogens like *Entamoeba histolytica*, *Giardia intestinalis*, and *Cryptosporidium spp*, which cause diarrhea-associated illnesses such as amoebiasis, giardiasis, and cryptosporidiosis [20, 21]. These infections disproportionately affect children under five, causing malnutrition, stunted growth, and anemia [17, 22].

Globally, the WHO estimates that over 835 million children live in areas with high parasite transmission rates, where these infections compromise cognitive development and overall health [22]. Beyond physical health, IPIs significantly impact productivity, quality of life, and socioeconomic stability [23].

3. *Giardia* spp.

Diarrhea is the second leading cause of global mortality after lower respiratory infections [24]. *Giardia* is a flagellated protozoan parasite that infects the small intestine, colonizing the gastrointestinal tracts of a wide range of hosts, including humans, domestic and wild mammals, and various bird species [7, 25]. Giardiasis, caused by the protozoan parasite *Giardia*, is a common diarrheal illness that infects the intestines. The disease is zoonotic and prevalent worldwide, affecting both developed and developing countries. While giardiasis can affect individuals of all ages, children are particularly susceptible [20]. Annually, the disease impacts over 280 million people globally [26]. Its prevalence ranges from 2.5 to 8.5% in developed nations and 21–33% in developing regions [21].

3.1 History

The discovery of *Giardia* dates back to 1681 when Antony van Leeuwenhoek first observed the parasite using a microscope to examine his stool [27–29]. In 1859, Vilém Dušan Lambl provided a more detailed description, naming it *Cercomonas intestinalis* [30]. Later, Battista Grassi identified it in rodents and called it *Dimorphus muris* in 1879 [31]. In the early 1880s, Johann Künstler named the genus *Giardia* after French zoologist Alfred Giard [32]. Over time, various names, including *Giardia intestinalis*, *Giardia duodenalis*, and *Giardia lamblia*, were proposed [31].

The twentieth century saw increasing recognition of *Giardia* as a pathogen. Charles Wardell Stiles linked it to diarrhea during World War I, observing that infected soldiers passed cysts, causing similar symptoms in laboratory animals [33]. By 1954, Robert Rendtorff provided clear evidence of its pathogenicity [34]. Research from the 1950s to the 1970s explored its morphology, life cycle, and prevalence. Significant advancements occurred from the 1980s to the 1990s with genetic studies, including ribosomal RNA sequencing, revealing its genetic diversity [31, 35]. In 1999, a vaccine called GiardiaVax was developed for pets, reducing symptoms and cyst output [36].

The 2000s brought genomic sequencing of *Giardia*, completed in 2007, providing insights into its biology and potential drug targets [37]. Advances in molecular biology during the 2010s improved the understanding of its pathogenicity [37]. By 2020, researchers focused on new diagnostic tools, vaccines, and treatments, including exploring medicinal plants for anti-Giardia properties [38].

3.2 Classification

Giardia is a single-celled eukaryote classified under the kingdom Protista. It belongs to the phylum Sarcomastigophora, subphylum Mastigophora, Class Zoomastigophora, and order Diplomonadida, characterized by flagella and two identical nuclei [30, 39–42].

3.3 *Giardia* species and genotypes

There are over 50 species of *Giardia*, but molecular tools like PCR have refined the classification to six main species (**Table 1**) [9, 30, 43]. *Giardia* is further classified

Species	Hosts	Morphology
G. intestinalis	Mammals, including humans, dogs, and some wild species	Teardrop-shaped with claw-shaped median bodies
G. agilis	Amphibians	Longer and slender than *G. intestinalis*, with a teardrop-shaped median body
G. ardeae	Herons and other birds	Similar to *G. intestinalis*
G. psittaci	Psittacine birds	Similar to *G. intestinalis*
G. muris	Rodents	Shorter and rounder than *G. intestinalis*, with a small rounded median body
G. microti	Rodents, voles, and muskrats	Similar to *G. intestinalis*

Table 1.
Assemblages and sub-assemblages of Giardia *and their hosts [6, 43].*

into eight genotypes (A–H), with A and B infecting humans and mammals, C and D affecting canines, E targeting livestock, F infecting felines, G found in rodents, and H in aquatic mammals [43–46].

4. *Giardia intestinalis*

4.1 Basic morphology and life cycle

Giardia intestinalis exists in two forms: trophozoites (disease-causing) (**Figure 1**) and cysts (infectious) (**Figure 2**) [49]. Trophozoites are pear-shaped, 9–21 μm long, with two nuclei, four pairs of flagella, and a ventral disc for intestinal adhesion (**Figure 1**) [47, 50, 51]. Cysts are ovoid, 12 × 6 μm in size, with four nuclei, and a thick protective wall, enabling survival in the environment [30, 50, 52].

The *Giardia intestinalis* life cycle alternates between the trophozoite and cyst stages (**Figure 3**) [54]. Infection begins with ingestion of cysts through contaminated food or water [55]. In the stomach, acidic conditions trigger excystation, releasing trophozoites, which colonize the small intestine and multiply [6, 54, 56]. In the lower portion of the small intestine, trophozoites undergo encystation and form cysts that are excreted in feces, remaining infectious in the environment [30, 54, 57].

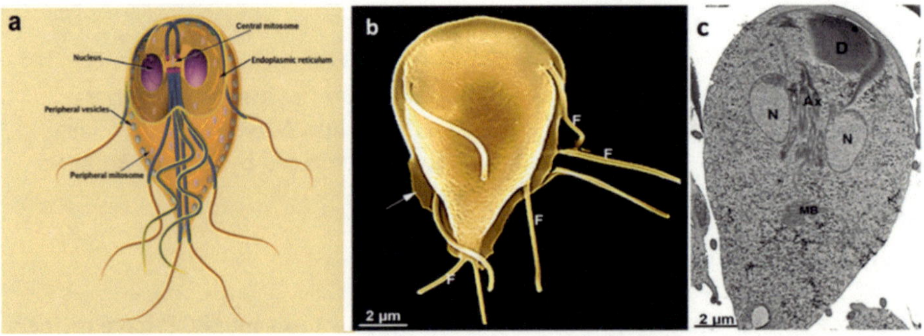

Figure 1.
G. intestinalis *trophozoite morphology, (a)* G. intestinalis *trophozoite, (b) scanning electron microscopy of the parasite, and (c) transmission electron microscopy of a trophozoite. Adapted from [47, 48].*

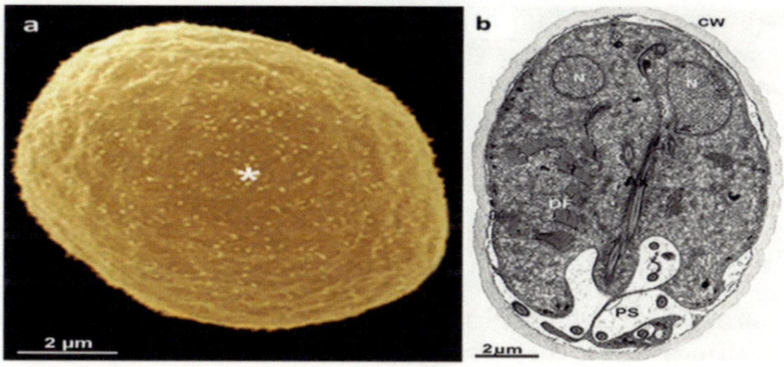

Figure 2.
G. intestinalis *cyst morphology (a)* G. intestinalis *cyst using scanning electron microscopy, and (b) transmission electron microscopy of a cyst. The nuclei (N), disc fragments (DF), and axonemes (Ax) are observed, as well as the cyst wall (CW) and peritrophic space (PS). Adapted from [47].*

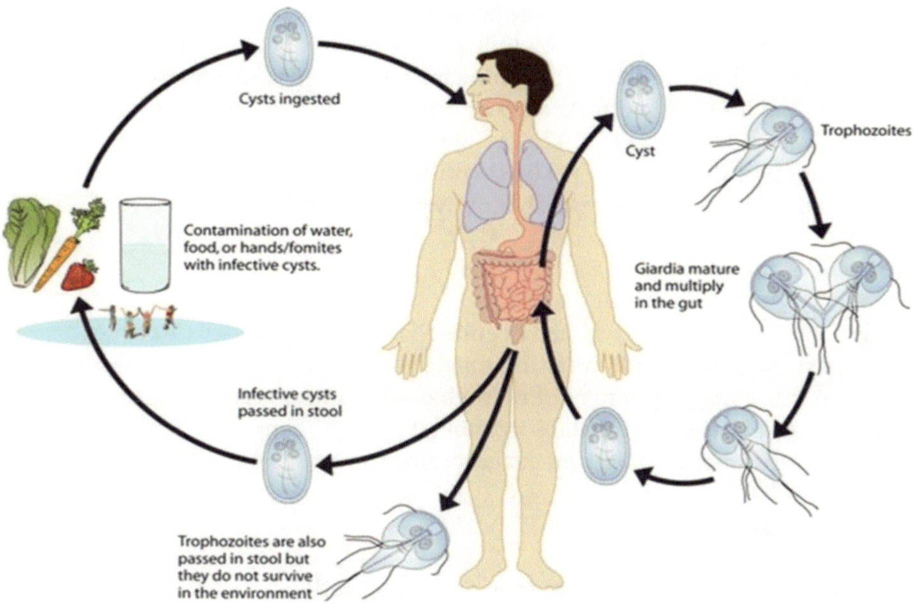

Figure 3.
Life cycle of G. intestinalis. *Adapted from [53].*

4.2 Genomics

Giardia intestinalis is about 12 Mb genome, organized into a diploid set of five chromosomes, 4863 protein-coding genes, and 306 pseudogenes [58–60]. It has a compact structure with minimal non-coding regions and includes microRNAs for gene regulation. Eight genotypes (assemblages A–H) have been identified [6, 60].

4.3 Metabolism

Giardia intestinalis lacks mitochondria and relies on glycolysis for ATP, though glucose is not its primary fuel [44, 60, 61]. It uses the arginine dihydrolase pathway for efficient energy production [44]. *Giardia* trophozoites rely on preformed lipids, while purines and pyrimidines are exclusively sourced from the host due to the parasite's inability to synthesize them [44, 60].

5. Giardiasis

5.1 Transmission

Giardia intestinalis is highly transmissible through various routes and poses significant challenges due to the persistence of its infectious cysts [62]. Transmission occurs *via* direct (person-to-person or zoonotic) or indirect (waterborne or food-borne) pathways [63].

5.2 Clinical manifestation

Infection with *G. intestinalis* can be asymptomatic in 60–80% of cases [19, 56]. When symptoms occur, they may include diarrhea, abdominal pain, bloating, weight loss, nausea, and fever [6, 64, 65]. Chronic infections can lead to malabsorption, steatorrhea, and long-term effects such as inflammatory bowel syndrome (IBS), arthritis, and cognitive issues [9, 12, 19, 56, 66]. Children are more prone to symptoms due to weaker immunity [63, 67]. The severity of symptoms depends on factors such as age, immune status, and the number of cysts ingested [19, 45].

5.3 Pathogenesis

G. intestinalis trophozoites attach to epithelial cells in the small intestine, disrupting the intestinal barrier and impairing nutrient absorption [19, 68]. This leads to increased permeability, apoptosis of epithelial cells, and shortening of microvilli, contributing to diarrhea and malabsorption [19]. Disruption of tight junctions further compromises the intestinal barrier, exacerbating the symptoms of giardiasis [51, 69].

5.4 Immune responses

The immune response to *G. intestinalis* involves both innate and adaptive immunity working together to combat the parasite [70].

5.4.1 Innate immunity

The first defense against infection is activated upon the parasite's contact with the intestinal epithelium. Macrophages, mast cells, and dendritic cells are involved in recognizing and responding to the pathogen [30, 44]. Producing pro-inflammatory cytokines to initiate immune responses. Nitric oxide plays a role in controlling parasite replication [70].

5.4.2 Adaptive immunity

T-cells (CD4+ and CD8+) are crucial in the response. CD4+ T-cells help activate B-cells and produce antibodies, while CD8+ T-cells eliminate infected cells [44, 70]. Cytokines, such as IL-17, TNF-α, and IFN-γ, help control the infection, whereas Th2 cytokines regulate inflammation [44, 71]. B-cells produce IgA antibodies, which play an important role in controlling G. intestinalis at mucosal sites [44, 70].

5.5 Prevalence

Giardiasis is more common in areas with poor sanitation and lack of clean water treatment [72]. It has been estimated that there are 280 million cases of giardiasis worldwide each year [56]. While prevalence rates of giardiasis range from 10 to 20%

Country	Host	N. of examined samples	Method of analysis	Prevalence	Ref.
UK	Human	212	Enzyme immunoassay (EIA)	41 (57%)	[74]
Russia	Dogs cats	1752 dogs and 1261 cats	Flotation and sedimentation techniques	172 dogs (9.8%) and 59 cats (4.6%)	[75]
Colombia	Dogs	100	Microscopic examination and PCR	47 (47%)	[76]
Qatar	Human	54	PCR	Assemblage A in 9 (16.67%), assemblage B in 30 (55.55%), and a mixture of assemblages A + B in 15 (27.78%)	[77]
Syria	Human	40	PCR	Assemblages A (67.5%), assemblages B (10%) and a mixed of assemblages A + B (22.5%).	[78]
Ethiopia	Human	422	Microscopic examination	27.1%.	[79]
Cuba	Human	417	Microscopic examination	45 (10.8%)	[80]
Algeria	Human	2054	Microscopic examination	97 (63.9%)	[81]
Nepal	Human	333	Microscopic examination and qPCR	63 (18.9%)	[82]
South Africa	Human	516	Immunological and molecular methods	40 (7.75%)	[83]
Korea	Calves	590	PCR and ELISA	77 (13.1%)	[84]
Mexico	Human	173	Faust technique	40 (23%)	[85]
Turkey	Dogs	473	Microscopic examination and PCR	18.80%	[86]
Ethiopia	Human	393	Real-time PCR	216 (55.0%)	[87]
Nigeria	Pigs	209	ELISA	53 (25.4%)	[88]
Italy	Dogs	168	Parasitological techniques and a rapid immunoassay	69(41%)	[89]
Saudi Arabia	Human	407	Microscopic examination	2%	[90]

Table 2.
Prevalence of Giardia *in some countries of the world.*

of the overall population, from 20 to 30% in impoverished countries, and from 3 to 7% in industrialized nations [49, 73].

Table 2 displays that various studies across different countries have reported different prevalence rates. The prevalence can vary depending on geographical location, urban or rural settings, age groups, hygiene, and socioeconomic factors [91]. Various epidemiological studies have reported different prevalence rates, suggesting that these rates may be greatly understated. This could be explained by the high percentage of asymptomatic carriers, who nevertheless aid in the spread of the illnesses even in the absence of symptoms [91].

5.6 Diagnosis

Diagnosing *G. intestinalis* infection is essential for effective treatment and prevention, though it can be challenging due to non-specific clinical symptoms [14, 92]. Several methods are used to detect the infection, including microscopy, immunodiagnostic tests, and molecular diagnostics [25, 92].

5.6.1 Microscopy examination

Microscopy is the most common method for diagnosing giardiasis by identifying cysts or trophozoites in stool samples [25]. This method is affordable and widely used, but it requires expertise and is not very sensitive for identifying different species [63, 93, 94]. Multiple stool samples may be needed because cysts are sometimes shed intermittently [14, 49].

5.6.2 Immunodiagnostic tests

Immunodiagnostic methods like ELISA and immunochromatographic tests are faster and more sensitive than microscopy [14, 94]. These tests detect antibodies against *G. intestinalis* in stool or serum, making them reliable for diagnosis [14]. However, they may give false-positive or false-negative results and are best used alongside microscopy [14, 95].

5.6.3 Molecular diagnostic

Molecular techniques, especially PCR, are the most sensitive and specific methods for detecting *G. intestinalis* [96]. PCR can detect the parasite's DNA in stool, blood, and saliva, allowing for accurate identification and molecular typing [93, 97, 98]. Although PCR is highly reliable, it can be expensive and requires skilled technicians [92].

5.7 Treatment

Despite recent reductions in the worldwide occurrence, giardiasis remains a serious public health concern due to the high number of cases that have been documented. This poses a risk of transmission and economic burdens [9, 61]. Giardiasis with symptoms should be treated to reduce the illness's symptoms, avoid complications, and prevent the parasite's ability to infect other hosts [11, 49]. Several drugs are currently recommended for treating giardiasis, reflecting the ongoing efforts to manage and combat this infection [9].

5.7.1 Chemotherapy treatment

Giardiasis is traditionally treated with chemotherapy using two groups of medications: benzimidazole derivatives (albendazole and mebendazole), nitroimidazole derivatives (metronidazole, tinidazole, secnidazole, and ornidazole), nitazoxanide, furazolidone, quinacrine, chloroquine, and paromomycin [9, 24, 44, 99].

Metronidazole has long been the first-line treatment, as it targets the DNA of the *Giardia* parasite, preventing it from replication [98, 100]. However, while effective in many cases, its use has been linked to adverse side effects [101]. Moreover, drug resistance in *Giardia* has been increasingly reported, which has made treatment less effective, especially in chronic and recurrent cases, with many cases refractory to metronidazole treatment. These can result from reinfection, inadequate drug dose, immunosuppression, and eventual *Giardia* sequestration in the gallbladder or the pancreatic duct [101].

Tinidazole, another chemotherapy option, offers the advantage of requiring only a single dose, which improves patient compliance, but similar resistance concerns have emerged [102].

5.7.2 Phytoproducts and nanotechnology as treatment agents

The emergence of drug resistance has led researchers to look for alternative treatments including the use of medicinal plants [99]. Many populations depend on medicinal herbs and their derivatives as cost-effective, accessible, and advantageous alternatives for treating a wide range of diseases [103]. Medicinal plants are considered important alternative sources for treating *Giardia* infections due to their potential to offer effective treatment with fewer side effects than other drugs [9]. Certain plants, like pomegranate (*Punica granatum*) and tansy (*Tanacetum vulgare*), have shown antimicrobial activity against *Giardia* comparable to metronidazole in laboratory settings [9, 104]. These plants could potentially provide additional treatment options, especially in areas where drug resistance is a concern or where access to pharmaceutical treatments is limited. However, further studies are needed to assess the safety and effectiveness of these plant-based treatments before they can be recommended for widespread use [105].

In addition to plant-based treatments, nanotechnology is emerging as a promising strategy for combating parasitic infections [106]. Nanoparticles, such as selenium and chitosan, have demonstrated enhanced anti-*Giardia* properties by improving drug absorption and targeting parasites more efficiently [107, 108]. Selenium nanoparticles, for example, have shown comparable efficacy to metronidazole with fewer side effects [107], while chitosan nanoparticles disrupt the parasite's cell wall, leading to its death [108]. These advancements in nanotechnology offer potential improvements in treatment effectiveness, suggesting that they could be employed as a safe, effective alternative therapy for giardiasis [108, 109].

5.8 Control and prevention of giardiasis

Giardiasis is treated with metronidazole, but some reports suggest the parasite may develop resistance to this drug [110]. Therefore, it is important to combine treatment with other prevention measures to lower general prevalence and transmission [110]. The main way for *Giardia* to spread is through contaminated water and food. To reduce this, it is crucial to keep water and food clean, wash hands regularly, and educate people about hygiene [11, 30, 49]. Infected people should avoid swimming in public pools to prevent the spreading of the parasite [30, 49]. Also, methods like boiling or filtering water can kill *Giardia* cysts [62, 92]. Animals can also help in giardiasis spread, so it is important to treat and wash animals regularly and maintain clean farm environments [92, 111].

5.9 Vaccination against giardiasis

Currently, there is no human vaccine for giardiasis [112]. Developing a vaccine is difficult because Giardia has a complex life cycle and can avoid the immune system. A vaccine for animals, called GiardiaVax, was developed but did not work for humans [36, 113, 114]. Some experimental vaccines target proteins on the surface of *Giardia* [115]. However, no vaccine is currently available for human use [112].

6. Conclusions

Giardiasis still poses a serious threat to world health, impacting both people and animals. This chapter has the main facets of the illness, such as prevention, treatment, and prospects, covered. Chemotherapy remains the primary treatment option, with metronidazole and tinidazole being used extensively; however, growing drug resistance highlights the urgent need for alternative therapeutic approaches. The potential of natural remedies and plant-based treatments has shown promise and offers promising alternatives, while advancements in vaccine development for humans could provide long-term solutions.

Conflict of interest

The authors declare no conflict of interest.

Author details

Haleema H. Albohiri[1], Eman S. Elwakil[2*], Sarah Albalawi[1] and Muslimah N. Alsulami[1]

1 Department of Biological Sciences, College of Science, University of Jeddah, Jeddah, Saudi Arabia

2 Department of Parasitology, Theodor Bilharz Research Institute, Giza, Egypt

*Address all correspondence to: e.el-wakil@tbri.gov.eg

References

[1] Krumrie S. Molecular epidemiology of *Giardia duodenalis* in the high-income world [PhD thesis]. University of Glasgow; 2022

[2] Nii-Trebi N. Emerging and neglected infectious diseases: Insights, advances, and challenges. BioMed Research International. 2017;**2017**(5245021):1-15

[3] Wolday D, Gebrecherkos T, Arefaine ZG, Kiros YK, Gebreegzabher A, Tasew G, et al. Effect of co-infection with intestinal parasites on COVID-19 severity: A prospective observational cohort study. EClinicalMedicine. 2021;**39**:101054. Available from:. DOI: 10.1016/j.eclinm.2021.101054

[4] Herricks JR, Hotez PJ, Wanga V, Coffeng LE, Haagsma JA, Basanez M-G, et al. The global burden of disease study 2013: What does it mean for the NTDs? PLoS Neglected Tropical Diseases. 2017;**11**(8):1-21

[5] Al-Malki JS. Prevalence and risk factors of parasitic diseases among Saudi children. Saudi Medical Journal. 2021;**42**(6):612-619

[6] Adam RD. *Giardia duodenalis*: Biology and pathogenesis. Clinical Microbiology Reviews. 2021;**34**(4):e00024-e00019

[7] Anderson A. The parasite *giardia* [undergraduate honors thesis]. University of Nebraska-Lincoln; 2020. pp. 1-17

[8] Fekete E, Sosnowski O, Buret AG. *Giardia Spp*. and the gut microbiota: Dangerous liaisons. Frontiers in Microbiology. 2021;**11**:618106

[9] Mureșan ML, Cozma-Petruț A, Benedec D, Revnic C, Hanganu D, Dinte E, et al. Anti-Giardia activity of Tanacetum Vulgare flowers extract on infected mice. Farmácia. 2021;**69**(6):1128-1132

[10] Riches A, Hart CJS, Trenholme KR, Skinner-Adams TS. Anti-Giardia drug discovery: Current status and gut feelings. Journal of Medicinal Chemistry. 2020;**63**(22):13330-13354

[11] Dixon BR. Giardia duodenalis in humans and animals – Transmission and disease. Research in Veterinary Science. 2021;**135**(September):283-289. Available from:. DOI: 10.1016/j.rvsc.2020.09.034

[12] Allain T, Fekete E, Sosnowski O, De LDD, Motta JP, Leger D, et al. High - fat diet increases the severity of Giardia infection in association with low - grade inflammation and gut microbiota dysbiosis. Scientific Reports. 2021;**0123456789**:1-17. Available from:. DOI: 10.1038/s41598-021-98262-8

[13] Cernikova L, Faso C, Hehl AB. Five facts about Giardia lamblia. PLoS Pathogens. 2018;**14**(9):e1007250

[14] Hooshyar H, Rostamkhani P, Arbabi M, Delavari M. Giardia lamblia infection: Review of current diagnostic strategies. Gastroenterology and Hepatology: Bench to Bedside. 2019;**12**(1):3-12

[15] Díaz VMM. Pharmacological treatment of giardiasis. In: Rodriguez AJ, editor. Current Topics in Giardiasis. London, UK: IntechOpen; 2017. pp. 133-145

[16] Mark Jourdan P, Helen Louise Lamberton P, Fenwick A, Addiss DG, Lamberton P. Soil-transmitted helminth infections in humans: Clinical

management and public health control. Lancet. 2018;**391**(10117):252-265. Available from: https://pubmed.ncbi.nlm.nih.gov/28882382/

[17] Sitotaw B, Mekuriaw H, Damtie D. Prevalence of intestinal parasitic infections and associated risk factors among Jawi primary school children, Jawi town, North-West Ethiopia. BMC Infectious Diseases. 2019;**19**(1):1-10

[18] Hailegebriel T. Prevalence of intestinal parasitic infections and associated risk factors among students at Dona Berber primary school, Bahir Dar, Ethiopia. BMC Infectious Diseases. 2017;**17**(1):1-8

[19] Faria C. Molecular Characterization of *Giardia lamblia* from Patients of a Referral Hospital of Rio de Janeiro/Brazil: Application of Multilocus Genotyping to Study the Inter and. 2017. Available from: https://estudogeral.sib.uc.pt/handle/10316/32153

[20] Dhakal N. Intestinal Parasites in Meche Community in Relation to their Socio-Economic Status. 2019.

[21] Kamonge S, Kamau L, Muhoho N. Prevalence of intestinal parasitic infections and transmission risk factors in primary school children in Mbeere north Sub-County, Embu County, Kenya. International Journal of Pathogen Research. 2020;**4**(3):1-7

[22] Chelkeba L, Mekonnen Z, Alemu Y, Emana D. Epidemiology of intestinal parasitic infections in preschool and school-aged Ethiopian children: A systematic review and meta-analysis. BMC Public Health. 2020;**20**(1):1-16

[23] Elmonir W, Elaadli H, Amer A, El-Sharkawy H, Bessat M, Mahmoud SF, et al. Prevalence of intestinal parasitic infections and their associated risk factors among preschool and school children in Egypt. PLoS One. 2021;**16**(9 September):1-11. DOI: 10.1371/journal.pone.0258037

[24] Enriquez V. Molecular and cellular characterizations of glucosylceramide transferase (synthase) in Giardia lamblia [PhD thesis]. The University of Texas at El Paso; 2021

[25] Chang Y, Li J, Zhang L. Genetic diversity and molecular diagnosis of Giardia. Infection, Genetics and Evolution. 2023;**113**(May):105482. DOI: 10.1016/j.meegid.2023.105482

[26] Pouryousef A, Fararouei MSB. Antigen-based diagnosis of human giardiasis: A systematic review and meta-analysis. 2023;**18**(2):140-154

[27] Ford BJ. The discovery of Giardia 1. 2005;**53**(September 2004):147-153

[28] Dobell C. The discovery of the intestinal protozoa of man. Proceedings of the Royal Society of Medicine. 1920;**13**(Sect_Hist_Med):1-15

[29] Steuart RFL, O'Handley R, Lipscombe RJ, Lock RA, Thompson RCA. Alpha 2 giardin is an assemblage A-specific protein of human infective Giardia duodenalis. Parasitology. 2008;**135**(14):1621-1627

[30] Seher M, Al-Kahfaji A, Alsaadi ZH. Giardia Lamblia and Giardiasis. Journal of University of Babylon for Pure and Applied Sciences. 2019;**27**:2019

[31] Adam RD. Biology of Giardia lamblia. Clinical Microbiology Reviews. 2001;**14**(3):447-475

[32] Dubourg A. Giardia trophozoite - Secreted Proteins and their effects on

intestinal epithelia [diss]. University of East Anglia; 2014

[33] Cox FEG. History of human parasitology. Clinical Microbiology Reviews. 2002;**15**(4):595-612

[34] Rendtorff RC, Holt CJ. The experimental transmission of human intestinal protozoan parasites. American Journal of Epidemiology. 1955;**61**(3):321-325

[35] Rayani M, Zasmy Unyah N, Hatam G. Molecular identification of Giardia duodenalis isolates from Fars Province, Iran. Iranian Journal of Parasitology. 2014;**9**(1):70-78

[36] Davids BJ, Liu CM, Hanson EM, Le CHY, Ang J, Hanevik K, et al. Identification of conserved candidate vaccine antigens in the surface proteome of *Giardia lamblia*. Infection and Immunity. 2019;**87**(6):10-1128

[37] Jerlström-Hultqvist J, Franzén O, Ankarklev J, Xu F, Nohýnková E, Andersson JO, et al. Genome analysis and comparative genomics of a Giardia intestinalis assemblage E isolate. BMC Genomics. 2010;**11**(1):1-15

[38] Bendtsen L, Zakrzewska JM, Heinskou TB, Hodaie M, Leal PRL, Nurmikko T, et al. Advances in diagnosis, classification, pathophysiology, and management of trigeminal neuralgia. Lancet Neurology. 2020;**19**(9):784-796. DOI: 10.1016/S1474-4422(20)30233-7

[39] Verma AK. Protozoans: Animals or protists. International Journal of Life Sciences. 2021;**9**(1):41-44

[40] Prykhodko A, Popovich A, Yemets T, Maleeva A. Molecular and Cellular Levels of Living Things Organization. Genetics: Zaporozhye State Medical University; 2016. pp. 1-135

[41] Adam RD, Archibald JM, Simpson AGB, Slamovits CH, Margulis L, Melkonian M, et al. Handbook of the Protists. 2nd ed. Cham: Springer International Publishing; 2017. pp. 1219-1246. Available from: https://link.springer.com/10.1007/978-3-319-32669-6

[42] David T, John MPD, William A, Petri MDPD, Martin G. Medical parasitology. In: Elsevier Health Sciences. 10th Sea ed. 2006. Available from: https://books.google.com.sa/books?id=O2n2DwAAQBAJ

[43] Gutiérrez AMQ. Giardiasis epidemiology. In: Current Topics in Giardiasis. London, UK: InTech; 2017. Available from: http://www.intechopen.com/books/current-topics-in-giardiasis/giardiasis-epidemiology

[44] Peirasmaki D. Studies of Giardia-host interactions: Role of cysteine-rich surface proteins [diss]. Acta Universitatis Upsaliensis; 2019

[45] Allain T, Buret AG. Pathogenesis and post-infectious complications in giardiasis. Advances in Parasitology. 2020;**107**:173-199

[46] Messa A, Köster PC, Garrine M, Gilchrist C, Bartelt LA, Nhampossa T, et al. Molecular diversity of Giardia duodenalis in children under 5 years from the manhiça district, southern Mozambique enrolled in a matched case-control study on the aetiology of diarrhoea. PLoS Neglected Tropical Diseases. 2021;**15**(1):1-24

[47] Benchimol M, Gadelha AP, de Souza W. Unusual cell structures and organelles in Giardia intestinalis and Trichomonas vaginalis are potential drug targets. Microorganisms. 2022;**10**(11):2176

[48] Midlej, Victor and Souza, Wanderley and Benchimol M. The Endomembrane

System of Giardia Intestinalis. London, UK: InTech; 2017. Available from: http://www.intechopen.com/books/current-topics-in-giardiasis/the-endomembrane-system-of-giardia-intestinalis

[49] Leung AKC, Leung AAM, Wong AHC, Sergi CM, Kam JKM. Giardiasis: An Overview. Recent Patents on Inflammation & Allergy Drug Discovery. 2019;**13**(2):134-143

[50] Benchimol M, Gadelha AP, de Souza W. Ultrastructural alterations of the human pathogen Giardia intestinalis after drug treatment. Pathogens. 2023;**12**(6):810. Available from: https://www.mdpi.com/2076-0817/12/6/810

[51] Rojas-López L, Marques RC, Svärd SG. Giardia duodenalis. Trends in Parasitology. 2022;**38**(7):605-606. Available from: https://linkinghub.elsevier.com/retrieve/pii/S1471492222000022

[52] Horton B. Identification of *Giardia duodenalis* in environmental and animal samples in Scotland with development of novel approaches of filtration elution [diss]. Heriot-Watt University; 2017. pp. 1-139

[53] Rawlings V. The role of dam water as a source of *Cryptosporidium* and *Giardia* infection in young sheep [Diss]. Murdoch University; 2018

[54] Fink MY, Shapiro D, Singer SM. Giardia lamblia: Laboratory maintenance, lifecycle induction, and infection of murine models. Current Protocols in Microbiology. 2020;**57**(1):1-22

[55] Horlock-Roberts K, Reaume C, Dayer G, Ouellet C, Cook N, Yee J. Drug-free approach to study the unusual cell cycle of Giardia intestinalis. mSphere. 2017;**2**(5):1-17. Available from: https://journals.asm.org/doi/10.1128/mSphere.00384-16

[56] Indieka R. Performance of one-step spanbio™ rapid test in detection of Giardia lamblia in Busia county referral hospital, western Kenya [diss]. Maseno University; 2022

[57] Rojas-lópez L. Regulation of differentiation during the *Giardia* life cycle: An insight into the molecular control [diss]. Acta Universitatis Upsaliensis; 2022

[58] Xu F, Jex A, Svärd SG. A chromosome-scale reference genome for Giardia intestinalis WB. Scientific Data. 2020;7(1):38. Available from: https://www.nature.com/articles/s41597-020-0377-y

[59] Xue M, Chen B, Ye Q, Shao J, Lyu Z, Wen J. Sense-antisense gene overlap is probably a cause for retaining the few introns in Giardia genome and the implications. Biology Direct. 2018;**13**(1):1-7

[60] Julia Walochnik MD. Molecular parasitology. In: Walochnik J, Duchêne M, editors. Scientist. Vol. 10. Vienna: Springer Vienna; 2016. Available from: http://link.springer.com/10.1007/978-3-7091-1416-2

[61] Hart CJ, Skinner-Adams T, Andrews KT, Ryan JH, Riches A. Identifying New Compounds Active against Giardia Duodenalis. Griffith University; 2020. DOI: 10.25904/1912/2113

[62] Feng C, Xu Z, Li Y, Zhu N, Wang Z. Research progress on the contamination status and control policy of Giardia and Cryptosporidium in drinking water. Journal of Water Sanitation and Hygiene for Development. 2021;**11**(6):867-886

[63] Dixon BR. Giardia duodenalis in humans and animals – Transmission and disease. Research in Veterinary Science. 2021;**135**(June):283-289. DOI: 10.1016/j.rvsc.2020.09.034

[64] Hikal WM. Parasitic contamination of drinking water and Egyptian standards for parasites in drinking water. Open Journal of Ecology. 2020;**10**(01):1-21

[65] Horton B, Bridle H, Alexander CL, Katzer F. Giardia duodenalis in the UK: Current knowledge of risk factors and public health implications. Parasitology. 2019;**146**(4):413-424

[66] Meningher T, Boleslavsky D, Barshack I, Tabibian-Keissar H, Kohen R, Gur-Wahnon D, et al. Giardia lamblia mirnas as a new diagnostic tool for human giardiasis. PLoS Neglected Tropical Diseases. 2019;**13**(6):1-16

[67] Thompson RCA, Ash A. Molecular epidemiology of Giardia and cryptosporidium infections. Infection, Genetics and Evolution. 2016;**40**:315-323. DOI: 10.1016/j.meegid.2015.09.028

[68] Certad G, Viscogliosi E, Chabé M, Cacciò SM. Pathogenic mechanisms of cryptosporidium and Giardia. Trends in Parasitology. 2017;**33**(7):561-576. DOI: 10.1016/j.pt.2017.02.006

[69] Solaymani-Mohammadi S. Mucosal defense against Giardia at the intestinal epithelial cell interface. Frontiers in Immunology. 2022;**13**(February):1-11

[70] Singer SM, Fink MY, Angelova VV. Recent insights into innate and adaptive immune responses to Giardia. In: Advances in Parasitology. 2019. pp. 171-208. Available from: https://linkinghub.elsevier.com/retrieve/pii/S0065308X19300314

[71] Serradell MC, Saura A, Rupil LL, Gargantini PR, Faya MI, Furlan PJ, et al. Vaccination of domestic animals with a novel oral vaccine prevents Giardia infections, alleviates signs of giardiasis and reduces transmission to humans. npj Vaccines. 2016;**1**(1):1-11

[72] Leder K, Weller DPF. Giardiasis: Epidemiology, Clinical Manifestations, and Diagnosis. UpToDate, Inc. and/or its affiliates. 2025. Available from: https://www.uptodate.com/contents/giardiasis-epidemiology-clinical-manifestations-and-diagnosis

[73] Mahdavi F, Sadrebazzaz A, Chahardehi AM, Badali R, Omidian M, Hassanipour S, et al. Global epidemiology of Giardia duodenalis infection in cancer patients: A systematic review and meta-analysis. International Health. 2022;**14**(1):5-17

[74] Waldram A, Vivancos R, Hartley C, Lamden K. Prevalence of Giardia infection in households of Giardia cases and risk factors for household transmission. BMC Infectious Diseases. 2017;**17**(1):486. Available from: http://bmcinfectdis.biomedcentral.com/articles/10.1186/s12879-017-2586-3

[75] Kurnosova OP, Arisov MV, Odoyevskaya IM. Intestinal parasites of pets and other house-kept animals in Moscow. Journal of Helminthology. 2019;**56**(2):108-117

[76] Hernández PC, Morales de la Pava L, Chaparro-Olaya J, López-Osorio S, López-Arias Á, Chaparro-Gutiérrez JJ. Multilocus genotyping of Giardia intestinalis in pet dogs of Medellín Colombia. 2021;**23**(131):100520

[77] Chourabi M, Boughattas S, Abdallah AM, Ismail A, Behnke JM, Al-Mekhlafi HM, et al. Genetic diversity and prevalence of Giardia duodenalis in

Qatar. Frontiers in Cellular and Infection Microbiology. 2021;**11**:652946

[78] Skhal D, Aboualchamat G, Al Mariri A, Al NS. Prevalence of Giardia duodenalis assemblages and sub-assemblages in symptomatic patients from Damascus city and its suburbs. Infection, Genetics and Evolution. 2017;**47**:155-160. DOI: 10.1016/j.meegid.2016.11.030

[79] Hajare ST, Chekol Y, Chauhan NM. Assessment of prevalence of Giardia lamblia infection and its associated factors among government elementary school children from Sidama zone, SNNPR, Ethiopia. PLoS One. 2022;**17**(3 March):1-17. DOI: 10.1371/journal.pone.0264812

[80] Puebla LJ, Núñez FA, García AB, Rivero LR, Millán IA, Prado RC. Prevalence of Giardia duodenalis among children from a central region of Cuba: Molecular characterization and associated risk factors. Journal of Parasitic Diseases. 2017;**41**(2):405-413

[81] Belkessa S, Ait-Salem E, Laatamna AE, Houali K, Sönksen UW, Hakem A, et al. Prevalence and clinical manifestations of Giardia intestinalis and other intestinal parasites in children and adults in Algeria. The American Journal of Tropical Medicine and Hygiene. 2021;**104**(3):910-916

[82] Tandukar S, Sherchand JB, Xue J, Uprety S, Sherchan SP, Bhandari D, et al. Prevalence and associated risk factors of Giardia duodenalis infection among school-going children in Nepal. Parasitology Research. 2018;**117**(1):287-293

[83] Samie A, Tanih NF, Seisa I, Seheri M, Mphahlele J, ElBakri A, et al. Prevalence and genetic characterization of Giardia lamblia in relation to diarrhea in Limpopo and Gauteng provinces, South Africa. Parasite Epidemiology and Control. 2020;**9**:e00140. DOI: 10.1016/j.parepi.2020.e00140

[84] Lee SH, VanBik D, Kim HY, Cho A, Kim JW, Byun JW, et al. Prevalence and molecular characterisation of Giardia duodenalis in calves with diarrhoea. The Veterinary Record. 2016;**178**(25):633

[85] Quihui-Cota L, Morales-Figueroa GG, Javalera-Duarte A, Ponce-Martínez JA, Valbuena-Gregorio E, López-Mata MA. Prevalence and associated risk factors for Giardia and Cryptosporidium infections among children of Northwest Mexico: A cross-sectional study. BMC Public Health. 2017;**17**(1):1-10

[86] Gultekin M, Ural K, Aysul N, Ayan A, Balikci C, Akyildiz G. Prevalence and molecular characterization of Giardia duodenalis in dogs in Aydin, Turkey. International Journal of Environmental Health Research. 2017;**27**(3):161-168. DOI: 10.1080/09603123.2017.1310187

[87] De Lucio A, Amor-Aramendía A, Bailo B, Saugar JM, Anegagrie M, Arroyo A, et al. Prevalence and genetic diversity of Giardia duodenalis and cryptosporidium spp. among school children in a rural area of the Amhara region, north-West Ethiopia. PLoS One. 2016;**11**(7):1-24

[88] Akinkuotu OA, Takeet MI, Otesile EB, Olufemi F, Greenwood SJ, McClure JT. Prevalence and mulilocus genotypes of Giardia duodenalis infecting pigs in Ogun state, Nigeria. Infection, Genetics and Evolution. 2019;**70**(January):53-60. DOI: 10.1016/j.meegid.2019.02.017

[89] Agresti A, Berrilli F, Maestrini M, Procesi IG, Loretti E, Vonci N, et al. Prevalence, risk factors and genotypes

of Giardia duodenalis in sheltered dogs in Tuscany (Central Italy). Pathogens. 2022;**11**(1):1-9

[90] Alshahrani M, Saif A, Bahnass M. Prevalence of intestinal parasitic infections among Saudis and expatriate workers in Najran, Saudi Arabia. The Zagazig Veterinary Journal. 2023;**51**(2):101-111

[91] Alemu Y, Abdissa A, Mekonnen Z, Sharew B, Johansen ØH, Bjørang O, et al. Prevalence and assemblage of Giardia duodenalis in a case-control study of children under 5 years from Jimma, Southwest Ethiopia. Parasitology Research. 2024;**123**(1):38

[92] Thigeel H. A study of factors associated with *Giardia* and *Cryptosporidiu*m infections in humans, dogs and cats in the USA [diss]. Colorado State University; 2016

[93] Rijsman LH, Monkelbaan JF, Kusters JG. Clinical consequences of polymerase chain reaction-based diagnosis of intestinal parasitic infections. Journal of Gastroenterology and Hepatology. 2016;**31**(11):1808-1815

[94] Soares R, Tasca T. Giardiasis: An update review on sensitivity and specificity of methods for laboratorial diagnosis. Journal of Microbiological Methods. 2016;**129**:98-102. Available from: https://linkinghub.elsevier.com/retrieve/pii/S016770121630224X

[95] Ryan U, Paparini A, Oskam C. New technologies for detection of enteric parasites. Trends in Parasitology. 2017;**33**(7):532-546. DOI: 10.1016/j.pt.2017.03.005

[96] Abbas AH, Bakhraibah AO, Al-Judaibi EA. An overview of the most recent studies on the prevalence of intestinal parasites among Saudi society, with an emphasis on expatriate workers. Microbial Biosystems. 2023;**8**(2):37-43

[97] O'Connell EM, Nutman TB. Review article: Molecular diagnostics for soil-transmitted helminths. The American Journal of Tropical Medicine and Hygiene. 2016;**95**(3):508-514

[98] Sanyang AM. Detection of Anti-*Giardia* Igg in Selected Orang Asli Serum Samples. University Sains Malaysia; 2019

[99] Santos HLC, Rebello KM. An overview of mucosa-associated protozoa: Challenges in chemotherapy and future perspectives. Frontiers in Cellular and Infection Microbiology. 2022;**12**(April):1-15

[100] Argüello-García R, Leitsch D, Skinner-Adams T, Ortega-Pierres MG. Drug resistance in Giardia: Mechanisms and alternative treatments for giardiasis. Advances in Parasitology. 2020;**107**:201-282

[101] Leitsch D. A review on metronidazole: An old warhorse in antimicrobial chemotherapy. Parasitology. 2019;**146**(9):1167-1178

[102] Ordóñez-Mena JM, McCarthy ND, Fanshawe TR. Comparative efficacy of drugs for treating giardiasis: A systematic update of the literature and network meta-analysis of randomized clinical trials. The Journal of Antimicrobial Chemotherapy. 2018;**73**(3):596-606

[103] Albalawi AE, Alanazi AD. Chemical composition, in vitro, and in vivo antiparasitic effects of Curcuma zedoaria rhizome essential oil against *Giardia lamblia*. Pharmacognosy Magazine. 2023;**19**(2):418-426. Available from: https://journals.sagepub.com/doi/10.1177/09731296231166055

[104] Elkholy WA, Elkholy MA, Elsokary AN, Alshehri E, Al-Quraishy S,

Abdel-Gaber R, et al. Therapeutic and prophylactic effects of *Punica granatum* peel extract versus metronidazole in murine giardiasis intestinalis. Journal of King Saud University - Science. 2022;**34**(8):102321. DOI: 10.1016/j.jksus.2022.102321

[105] Alnomasy S, Al-Awsi GRL, Raziani Y, Albalawi AE, Alanazi AD, Niazi M, et al. Systematic review on medicinal plants used for the treatment of Giardia infection. Saudi Journal of Biological Sciences. 2021;**28**(9):5391-5402. DOI: 10.1016/j.sjbs.2021.05.069

[106] Sundar S, Singh B. Emerging Therapeutic Targets for Treatment of Leishmaniasis. 2019;**22**(6):467-486

[107] Nikam PB, Salunkhe JD, Minkina T, Rajput VD, Soo B, Patil SV. Results in chemistry a review on green synthesis and recent applications of red nano selenium. Results in Chemistry. 2022;**4**(July):100581. DOI: 10.1016/j.rechem.2022.100581

[108] El-Gendy AML, Mohammed MAA, Ghallab MMI, Abdel Aziz MO, Ibrahim SM. Therapeutic effect of chitosan nanoparticles and metronidazole in treatment of experimentally giardiasis infected hamsters. Iranian Journal of Parasitology. 2021;**16**(1):32-42

[109] Yarahmadi M, Fakhar M, Ebrahimzadeh MA, Chabra A, Rahimi-esboei B. The anti-giardial effectiveness of fungal and commercial chitosan against Giardia intestinalis cysts in vitro. Journal of Parasitic Diseases. 2016;**40**(1):75-80. DOI: 10.1007/s12639-014-0449-z

[110] Archer J, O'Halloran L, Al-Shehri H, Summers S, Bhattacharyya T, Kabaterine NB, et al. Intestinal schistosomiasis and giardiasis co-infection in sub-Saharan Africa: Can a one health approach improve control of each waterborne parasite simultaneously? Tropical Medicine and Infectious Disease. 2020;**5**(3):1-20

[111] Santin M. Cryptosporidium and Giardia in ruminants. Veterinary Clinics of North America: Food Animal Practice. 2020;**36**(1):223-238. DOI: 10.1016/j.cvfa.2019.11.005

[112] Sangkanu S, Paul AK, Chuprom J, Mitsuwan W, Boonhok R, de Lourdes PM, et al. Conserved candidate antigens and nanoparticles to develop vaccine against Giardia intestinalis. Vaccine. 2023;**11**(1):96

[113] Vivancos V, González-Alvarez I, Bermejo M, Gonzalez-Alvarez M. Giardiasis: Characteristics, pathogenesis and new insights about treatment. Current Topics in Medicinal Chemistry. 2018;**18**(15):1287-1303

[114] Zhou J, Miyamoto Y, Ihara S, Kroll AV, Nieskens N, Tran VN, et al. Codelivery of antigens and adjuvant in polymeric nanoparticles coated with native parasite membranes induces protective mucosal immunity against *Giardia lamblia*. The Journal of Infectious Diseases. 2022;**226**(2):319-323

[115] Serradell MC, Gargantini PR, Saura A, Oms SR, Rupil LL, Berod L, et al. Cytokines, antibodies, and histopathological profiles during Giardia infection and variant-specific surface protein-based vaccination. Infection and Immunity. 2018;**86**(6):10-1128

Chapter 5

Perspective Chapter: Infectious Disease Surveillance in Urban Cities

Danish Nasar Khan and Aliya Rizvi

Abstract

The twenty-first century's unprecedented urban growth has fundamentally reshaped public health, creating unique challenges for disease surveillance in densely populated, dynamic urban environments. This chapter explores the critical need for robust urban disease surveillance and showcases innovations and best practices from global and Indian contexts. It emphasizes that an effective surveillance system must be capable of observing, monitoring, and responding to outbreaks to minimize their societal impact. Urban centers must evolve their systems to be smarter, more inclusive, and integrated with other areas like urban planning and digital infrastructure. The chapter details key innovations, including the use of digital health platforms, big data analytics, and AI for real-time data collection and analysis, as seen in systems like the U.S. CDC's BioSense and WHO's Epidemic Intelligence from Open Sources (EIOS). It also highlights the growing importance of community-oriented participatory surveillance, mobile applications, and wearable technologies for early detection and contact tracing. In the Indian context, the Integrated Disease Surveillance Programme (IDSP) has been a cornerstone, enhanced by digitalization and technologies like the Aarogya Setu app. Additionally, the chapter delves into core areas for strengthening urban surveillance: wastewater and environmental surveillance, outbreak response strategies, syndromic surveillance, entomological surveillance, urban slum surveillance, and private sector involvement. It provides a prescriptive roadmap for building resilient urban health surveillance by strengthening infrastructure, enhancing human resources, establishing strong policy frameworks, and fostering global and local collaboration. Ultimately, the effectiveness of twenty-first-century urban disease surveillance will depend on a combination of technology, community participation, and supportive policies.

Keywords: urban surveillance, health system strengthening, wastewater surveillance, entomological surveillance, disease surveillance, syndromic surveillance

1. Introduction

The twenty-first century is marked by unprecedented urban growth, fundamentally reshaping the public health landscape. As urban populations expand—projected to make up nearly 68% of the global total by 2050—the dynamics of disease transmission, detection, and control have undergone significant transformations. Urban environments, characterized by dense populations, mobile communities, informal settlements, and diverse health ecosystems, present unique challenges for public health governance. However, these very attributes also foster innovation and adaptive systems.

Urban disease surveillance has emerged as a cornerstone of public health preparedness and response. It represents the systematic collection, analysis, interpretation, and dissemination of health data specific to urban populations, geared toward early detection and containment of infectious and noninfectious diseases alike. In light of increasingly frequent public health emergencies—from pandemics to environmental hazards—surveillance systems in urban areas must evolve to become smarter, more inclusive, and deeply integrated with other domains such as urban planning, environmental monitoring, and digital infrastructure.

This chapter explores the imperative of urban disease surveillance by tracing historical developments, analyzing global and national best practices, and unpacking the institutional, technological, and societal levers that drive effective surveillance systems. Drawing heavily from a compendium of global best practices, the chapter aims to present not just a descriptive overview but also a prescriptive roadmap for building resilient urban health surveillance in a rapidly urbanizing world.

1.1 Bridging gaps in urban surveillance

Currently, disease surveillance in metropolitan areas relies heavily on the public sector, with limited private sector involvement, even though private providers deliver primary healthcare to approximately 70% of urban households (National Family Health Survey-3). The surveillance unit addresses this disparity by integrating private healthcare providers into the surveillance framework and enhancing reporting and analysis mechanisms. They also focus on vulnerable urban populations, such as those in slums and informal settlements, to ensure equitable health monitoring.

1.2 Need for strengthening urban surveillance

The COVID-19 pandemic has underscored the critical need for robust disease surveillance, particularly in metropolitan areas. These urban areas face unique challenges, including high population density, inadequate water and sanitation facilities, and rapid urban development, all of which elevate the risk of epidemics. Further, the unplanned urbanization in the metropolitan areas poses a major challenge in disease surveillance as compared to the suburban and rural areas.

The surveillance units are designed to fill the gaps in urban disease surveillance by targeting specific vulnerabilities: high density, poor sanitation, migrant populations, and extensive domestic and international travel. They aim to strengthen urban disease surveillance to meet the distinct health risks of the city by supplementing the resources and capacities of the existing IDSP for faster outbreak detection and response. The surveillance strategy of the Integrated Disease Surveillance Program through the district surveillance unit is not adequate to address the needs and challenges of metropolitan cities. Presently, the reporting is based mainly on the public sector, with only a limited involvement of the private sector. Seventy percent of urban households receive their primary healthcare from the private medical sector, according to the National Family Health Survey-3.

Hence, the review of the best practices on urban disease surveillance will help in implementing the innovations in the urban areas through the surveillance unit.

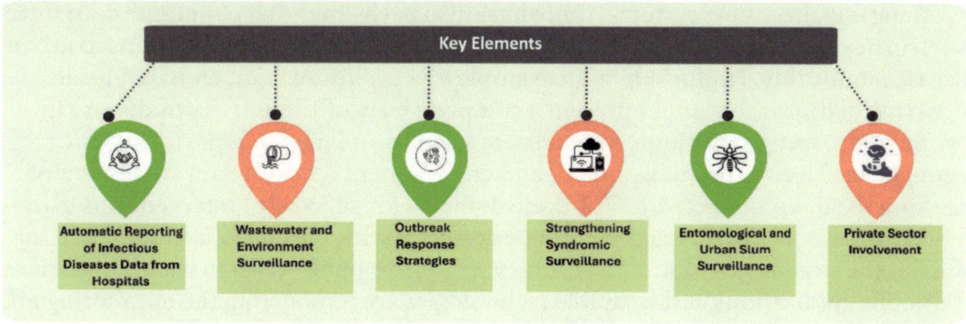

Figure 1.
Thematic area of urban surveillance.

This document will compile learnings from the global and Indian best practices in disease surveillance in the urban setting and improve the disease reporting with the available resources and settings.

1.3 Core areas related to the strengthening of urban disease surveillance

These are the key elements of urban disease surveillance (**Figure 1**).

2. Overview of the disease surveillance in an urban setting

Urban disease surveillance is a cornerstone of modern public health systems, particularly in densely populated cities where diseases can spread rapidly. Deriving from the high population density, dynamic movement of people, and interconnectivity, the urban area becomes a vulnerable area for disease outbreaks. An effective surveillance system should be able to observe, monitor, and respond to outbreaks so that the impacts on health and society can be reduced. This chapter showcases the innovations in urban disease surveillance in the global and Indian contexts, providing a holistic view of best practices and recommendations for strengthening these systems.

Globally, the landscape of digital health platforms for disease surveillance has altered, as it now permits the real-time collection, aggregation, and analysis of data. For example, *BioSense* by the U.S. Centers for Disease Control and Prevention (CDC) aggregates health data from multiple other sources to hasten the identification of outbreaks. The World Health Organization's Epidemic Intelligence from Open Sources *(EIOS)* exemplifies artificial intelligence *(AI)* in action, processing enormous quantities of data drawn from numerous sources, such as news reports and social media, for the purpose of discovering likely threats to public health. The increase in the use of digital technologies will, therefore, lead to better tracking and more informed decisions about diseases.

In fact, big data analytics and AI are still evolving in their roles regarding predictions and responses to diseases. A good example among many possibilities is Google's Flu Trends, which analyzes search engine data and can estimate flu activity. Following South Korea's lead in installing AI-powered *chatbots* to monitor COVID-19 symptoms and provide health advice, these powerful algorithms increase the speed and accuracy of data analysis. With these advances, health authorities will be in a position to discern trends, anticipate outbreaks, and optimally deploy resources.

Alongside these new systems, there have also been emerging community-oriented participatory disease surveillance systems that have been valuable additions to urban disease monitoring. *HealthMap* is an example of a traditional citizen-based health reporting platform that could present a complete view of the activity of disease in a population, using traditional surveillance systems and citizen reports. In Africa, through One Health, human, animal, and environmental health data are integrated, marking the interconnectedness of these domains for successful interventions to prevent outbreaks. By involving communities directly with the collection and reporting of data, the systems provide data accuracy and foster public trust in health initiatives.

Mobile applications and wearable technologies are remodeling the monitoring and management of diseases. An example that shows how mobile technologies are effective in tracking the mode of spread of diseases is the *TraceTogether* app by Singapore, specifically for contact tracing of COVID-19. The continuous measurement of physiological parameters such as heart rate and temperature helps wearables deliver real-time insight into the health of individuals and the public, thereby enabling early detection of everything from infectious diseases to chronic illnesses.

Another key feature of effective urban disease surveillance is interagency collaboration. The European Centre for Disease Prevention and Control *(ECDC)* is an example of how multiple jurisdictions working together can produce greater efficiencies in disease monitoring. It encourages the sharing of data on diseases and joint action among EU member states, thereby enhancing the collective ability to respond to health threats across borders.

In India, urban disease surveillance has witnessed significant advancements through innovative programs and technologies. The Integrated Disease Surveillance Programme *(IDSP)* is intended to become the bedrock of the Indian district-based surveillance outbreak detection and response effort. By digitalizing tools and services such as mobile applications and online reporting systems, the IDSP enhanced data collection and analysis. *Aarogya Setu* emerged as a key instrument in the country for contact tracing, symptom reporting, and health advisories during the COVID-19 pandemic, proving India's ability to swiftly employ technology for crisis situations.

The municipal health monitoring systems of cities, such as Mumbai and Bengaluru, are dealing with vector-borne diseases like dengue and chikungunya. Digital dashboards are used for case tracking, hotspot identification, and resource allocation. Surveillance has been boosted further by public-private partnerships *(PPPs)* with technology firms. For example, collaborations with startups that offer solutions driven by AI have further enhanced the prediction and monitoring of trends for diseases against proactive interventions.

Geospatial technology is a vital technology in the area of urban disease surveillance in India. GIS mapping is used to identify and predict disease hotspots. Integrating health data into urban planning involves projects such as Smart City initiatives. A good example of such an initiative is Bhubaneshwar's *Smart City project*, where geospatial tools can work to improve resource allocation and public health outcomes. Community engagement programs would also be vital, which include NGOs and health workers. Initiatives such as these sharpen awareness and promote participatory surveillance and thus empower citizens to take part more actively in public health.

To scale the innovations, one fundamentally starts from the base. Such steps may involve strengthening infrastructural investments, including cloud-based storage and processing systems for real-time access and reliability of data, and equipping health workers through regular training on digital tools and data interpretation. These, however, necessitate the establishment of strong policy frameworks guaranteeing data privacy while fostering inter- and intra-sectoral linkages. Public awareness communities could mobilize citizens toward disease case notification and uptake of surveillance technologies. On the other hand, global collaboration ensures that successful models are adapted to local contexts and thus will promote continuous improvement of the surveillance systems.

The urban centers will need to create a set of piloting examples that can kick-start the integration of global and local innovations into their local initiatives directed toward building a robust public health system for new health threats. It transforms what might be learning lessons from best practices into a seemingly short, real roadmap for strengthening disease surveillance and public health in urban settings. The effectiveness of urban disease surveillance will hinge on the triad of technology, community involvement, and policy support in the twenty-first century.

3. Automatic reporting of infectious disease data from hospitals

3.1 Brief background of the topic

A robust reporting system is a prerequisite for a surveillance system. By enabling early detection of emerging infectious diseases through near-real-time data collection, reducing delays caused by manual reporting processes, and ultimately resulting in better disease control and prevention strategies, automatic reporting of infectious disease data from hospitals is essential for enabling rapid public health response to outbreaks, improving disease surveillance accuracy, and facilitating timely interventions.

3.2 Summary of the literature

3.2.1 Real-time surveillance of infectious diseases: Taiwan's experience

In this program, the "communicable disease control cloud" performs automatic reporting using hospital electronic medical records (EMRs) [1].

Taiwan has a comprehensive network of laboratory, epidemiologic, and early-warning surveillance systems with nationwide representation. Hospitals and clinical laboratories have deployed automatic reporting mechanisms since 2014 and have effectively improved the timeliness of infectious disease and laboratory data reporting.

The National Notifiable Diseases System (NNDSS) of the Taiwan Centers for Disease Control (Taiwan CDC) has been the foundation of web-based infectious disease surveillance in Taiwan since 2001.

EMRs, because of the automatically integrated system to generalize patient-centered information, have reduced the average time required for a healthcare worker to complete the report process to the Taiwan CDC from 9.2 to 6.3 minutes.

Leveraging EMRs used in the private sector healthcare facilities for understanding infectious disease trends and implementing control measures.

The NEDSS (National Electronic Disease Surveillance System Base System) is a CDC-developed integrated information system that helps public health departments manage disease data and send it to the CDC. NEDSS helps public health agencies accept electronic data exchanges from healthcare systems and enables health departments to create and send standards-based case notifications to CDC for NNDSS.

Key highlights and strategic recommendations: IDSP is a flagship National Health Program mandated with disease surveillance of epidemic-prone diseases across 36 states/UTs through a decentralized structure. The data is captured through the Integrated Health Information Platform (IHIP), which is a case-based, near-real-time reporting platform for disease conditions and outbreaks. Integration of the IHIP with the EMR system of the health facilities and automatic reporting of infectious disease data from hospitals will revolutionize the surveillance mechanism.

4. Wastewater surveillance

In a world where early detection of disease outbreaks is critical to saving lives, researchers and public health officials have found a new ally in an unlikely place—wastewater. According to the implementation framework of NUHM (2001), the major deaths are reported by respiratory infections of about 16.5%, so the result is that the detection of airborne infection should be early. From the bustling cities of the United States to the distant corners of sub-Saharan Africa, wastewater-based epidemiology (WBE) is proving to be a revolutionary tool in the fight against infectious diseases. By analyzing pathogens shed into wastewater by individuals, both symptomatic and asymptomatic, WBE offers a noninvasive and cost-effective method to monitor the health of entire communities. This review explores the evolution of wastewater surveillance systems, their applications in detecting multiple pathogens, and the strategic recommendations for enhancing these systems.

4.1 Wastewater as a health sentinel

It all began with the establishment of the National Wastewater Surveillance System (NWSS) by the U.S. Centers for Disease Control and Prevention (CDC), which set the foundation for this pioneering public health strategy. The NWSS utilized wastewater to monitor the prevalence of infectious diseases such as SARS-CoV-2, influenza, and respiratory syncial virus (RSV). The system's success is grounded in its ability to capture data not just from symptomatic individuals but from entire communities, including those who might not seek healthcare. Through wastewater, the system detected early-warning signs of disease outbreaks, allowing public health authorities to allocate resources efficiently and implement targeted interventions [2].

Wastewater surveillance represents an invaluable tool in communities where traditional clinical surveillance falls short, either due to underreporting or lack of healthcare access. By integrating this method into the broader public health system, the NWSS helps paint a more complete picture of a community's health, one that includes the invisible, asymptomatic cases that often evade clinical detection (**Figure 2**).

4.2 The multiplex RT-qPCR revolution

In the field of pathogen detection, technology has continuously advanced, making systems like NWSS even more effective. One such breakthrough is the development of the multiplex RT-qPCR assay, which can simultaneously detect multiple viruses from wastewater samples. This technological innovation allows for the detection of viruses like SARS-CoV-2, influenza A, RSV, and even measles, all at once [3]. Prior methods required separate tests for each pathogen, making the process time-consuming and expensive. However, with multiplex RT-qPCR, the detection limits have improved

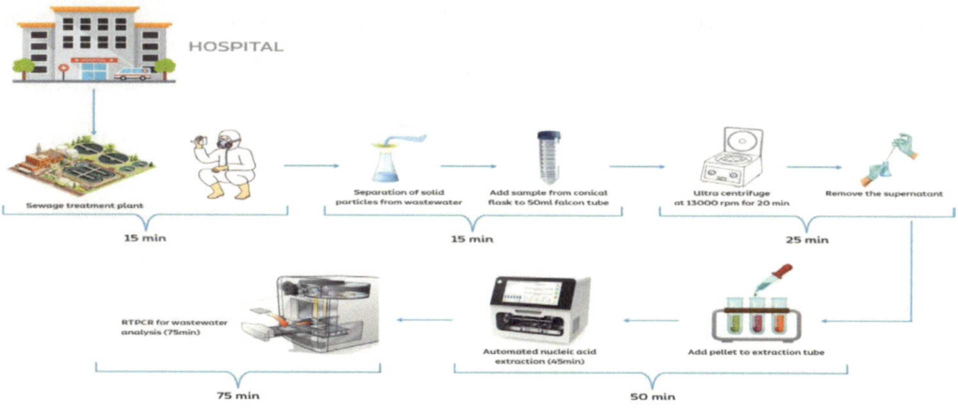

Figure 2.
Schematic diagram for the wastewater surveillance from the hospital sewage treatment plan.

significantly, with the assay achieving a sensitivity capable of detecting as few as 15–25 gene copies per reaction. This breakthrough means that wastewater surveillance can now detect viral ribose nucleic acid (RNA) weeks before clinical cases are reported, making it a powerful early-warning tool for pandemics and seasonal outbreaks.

The research demonstrates the robustness of the multiplex assay in various environmental conditions, even overcoming the inhibitors present in wastewater. Moreover, the system is more cost-effective than traditional methods, which makes it feasible for large-scale, ongoing surveillance. The ability to monitor multiple pathogens simultaneously with high sensitivity could dramatically enhance global pandemic preparedness and response [4].

4.3 Global expansion and broader applications

Wastewater-based epidemiology is not confined to the detection of respiratory viruses like COVID-19 or influenza. The application of WBE spans a wide range of pathogens, including gastrointestinal bacteria, protozoa, and even tuberculosis (TB). For example, a study conducted in Incheon, South Korea, tested treated wastewater for a variety of pathogens, including norovirus, hepatitis A, and Giardia lamblia. The results underscored the power of WBE to detect pathogens that affect different parts of the human body, not just the respiratory system [4].

Meanwhile, the focus has also shifted toward tuberculosis (TB), a disease that remains a significant public health challenge in many parts of Africa. In a groundbreaking study spanning six African countries—Ghana, Nigeria, Kenya, Uganda, Cameroon, and South Africa—researchers explored the potential of WBE to detect Mycobacterium tuberculosis complex (MTBC) in wastewater. The findings revealed that MTBC, which causes tuberculosis, was present in wastewater samples across all six countries, highlighting the utility of WBE as a tool for TB surveillance in regions with limited healthcare access [5].

4.4 The one health approach

One of the most intriguing aspects of WBE is its alignment with the One Health approach—a concept that recognizes the interconnectedness of human, animal, and environmental health. The detection of pathogens like MTBC in wastewater not only reveals community-level health trends but also raises concerns about environmental transmission. In Africa, where TB is prevalent, the detection of MTBC in treated wastewater calls attention to the potential risks of environmental transmission, which could affect downstream populations [2].

This idea of interconnected health systems is further reinforced by the discovery of seasonal trends in pathogen prevalence, as seen in the study from Incheon. Hepatitis A was found to peak during certain months, reflecting environmental factors that may influence disease transmission [4]. By monitoring the prevalence of various pathogens through WBE, public health officials can gain insights into seasonal patterns and develop more targeted interventions.

4.5 Strategic recommendations for strengthening wastewater-based epidemiology (WBE)

While the potential of WBE is vast, there are several steps that can further enhance its effectiveness in global health surveillance. First, it is crucial to *expand surveillance networks* to include underserved populations and regions with limited healthcare access. This expansion can help identify disease outbreaks early, especially in areas where clinical surveillance may be inadequate.

Second, developing *standardized protocols* for sampling and analysis is essential to ensure consistency and reliability across studies. This standardization would make it easier to compare data from different regions and ensure that the data collected is of the highest quality.

Third, integrating WBE into *existing public health systems* will enable real-time outbreak management. By combining data from clinical, environmental, and wastewater surveillance, health authorities can more effectively respond to emerging threats. *Investing in infrastructure* for wastewater treatment and genetic analysis will also improve the quality of data collected and enable faster responses.

Lastly, WBE's utility in tracking *high-impact pathogens* such as SARS-CoV-2, norovirus, and tuberculosis should be prioritized. The ability to detect these pathogens in wastewater allows for more proactive responses, helping to prevent large-scale outbreaks before they spread.

4.6 A new era in public health surveillance

Wastewater-based epidemiology has revolutionized how we think about public health monitoring. By providing a snapshot of disease prevalence in real time, WBE offers a powerful tool for early detection, outbreak management, and resource allocation. As technology continues to improve and more regions adopt these systems, WBE will undoubtedly become an integral part of global health surveillance, bridging the gaps left by traditional methods and providing a more holistic view of community health.

5. Environmental surveillance

Rapid urbanization has indisputably brought about sweeping changes to the socioeconomic landscape of India. However, it also brought with it a host of health-related issues. Today, cities are prevalent with bad air quality, increased susceptibility to zoonotic diseases, and constant healthcare-associated infections (HAIs). An example of an air quality crisis manifests in Delhi, which demonstrates how vehicular emissions, industrial discharges into the atmosphere, and agricultural practices such as stubble burning contribute to dangerous pollution levels [6]. This pollution is directly associated with respiratory and cardiovascular illnesses, specifically premature deaths that number high in India owing to air pollution every year [6]. The city's environmental health is further complicated by urban ecosystems that facilitate zoonotic and vector-borne diseases due to dense populations, climate variability, and poor infrastructure [7]. Simultaneously, the urban area has hospitals that are crowded and resource-constrained, and it is also a potential point for the establishment of hospital-acquired infections (HAIs), which are aggravated by the inconsistency of cleaning and increased microbial resistance [8]. This review aims to provide a strategic framework for relating environmental health, disease surveillance, and infection control in urban areas in India, based on previous works on air pollution in Delhi, environmental monitoring for infectious disease control, and multimodal approaches to infection prevention in hospitals.

5.1 Lesson learned

The COVID-19 lockdown provided a rare opportunity to observe the potential for air quality improvement in Delhi, with significant reductions in pollution levels achieved through decreased vehicular and industrial activities [6]. This emphasizes the potency of emission control policies as targeted in their application. Likewise, the incorporation of environmental matters such as precipitation trends together with vector observation has proven useful in anticipating outbreaks of diseases transmitted by mosquitoes [7]. This proves challenging because of the lack of funds and the expertise to institute such a monitoring framework in all cities [7]. In the domain of infection control, hospitals adopting bundled cleaning and disinfection strategies have reported notable reductions in HAIs, demonstrating the importance of consistent and evidence-based practices supported by government funding and monitoring [8].

5.2 Key urban health challenges

Pollution within the air is one of the major threats that could bring about an urban health crisis in the present time. Delhi, being one of the most polluted cities in the world, itself speaks much about the disease it carries with it. Chronic exposure to air pollutants in the form of particulate matter (PM2.5 and PM10) leads to various health problems, such as "asthma, bronchitis, lung cancer, and heart disease [6]." Current policies under the National Clean Air Program (NCAP) lack enforceable targets and accountability mechanisms and have not been framed to overcome cross-boundary pollution as well as the emissions from vehicles and industries that aggravate the pollution problem [6]. Additionally, India's urban landscapes are breeding grounds for zoonotic and vector-borne diseases, with climate variability such as altered rainfall patterns fueling the proliferation of vectors like mosquitoes [7]. Diseases such as dengue and malaria find a conducive environment in unchecked urban sprawl, which lacks standardized data collection for effective outbreak prediction [7]. Compounding these challenges are HAIs, which impose a significant burden on urban healthcare systems. Poorly maintained hospital environments, limited training of healthcare staff, and inconsistent application of cleaning strategies contribute to the persistence of pathogens and high morbidity rates [8].

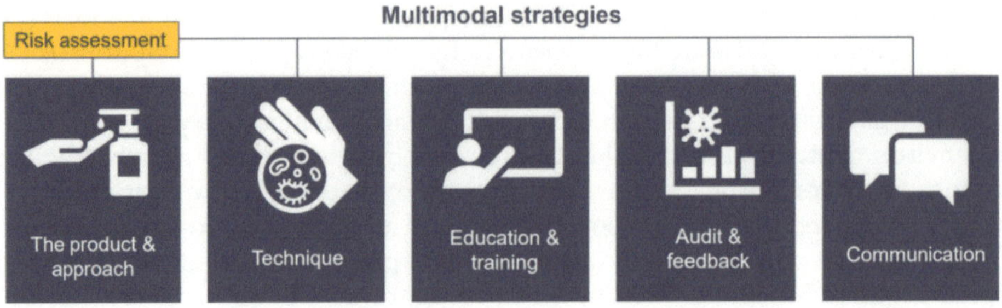

Figure 3.
*Multimodal strategy to combat hospital-acquired infections (*Courtesy: Browne, and Mitchell [8]*).*

5.3 Strategic recommendations for urban health surveillance

Strengthening environmental monitoring is essential for tackling urban health challenges. A robust framework that combines satellite data, IoT-enabled sensors, and local air quality indices can provide real-time insights into environmental health [7]. Such systems should be integrated with hospital infection records to enable predictive analytics that inform public health responses [8]. Comprehensive policy interventions are also necessary, with the expansion of the NCAP to include explicit health-focused goals and the establishment of an Urban Health Surveillance Authority (UHSA) to oversee disease monitoring and outbreak response [6, 7]. Advanced infection control practices, such as the adoption of multimodal cleaning strategies, regular training, and the use of technologies like UV-C disinfection, are crucial for reducing HAIs in urban healthcare facilities [8]. Leveraging technology, including AI-driven predictive models and mobile health apps, can empower citizens and authorities alike to monitor and respond to health risks effectively [7]. Community engagement through public awareness campaigns and collaborative governance can further enhance urban health resilience by fostering partnerships among municipal bodies, healthcare providers, and environmental agencies (**Figure 3**) [7].

The effects of air pollution, communicable diseases, and hospital-acquired infections thus pose a grave threat to India's urban health systems. Storming the storm by gushing environmental surveillance, strengthening policy frameworks, and adopting innovative practices in the healthcare system would develop resilient urban health ecosystems in India. The efforts should be strongly supported by the collaborative participation of all stakeholders—government, healthcare, and community—in order to create a healthier urban future. Goal-oriented, technology-driven solutions and collaborative community engagements with focused interventions are the crux to address health challenges in the urban system and set a global benchmark in public health resilience for the twenty-first century.

6. Outbreak response strategies

6.1 Brief background of the topic

Epidemic-prone communicable diseases remain a problem for public health systems worldwide, regardless of advancements in diagnosis and control techniques. Emerging and re-emerging diseases are among these circumstances, which could jeopardize the security of public health as well as financial and social benefits. Emerging and re-emerging diseases like cholera, dengue, H5N1 influenza, H1N1 influenza, Nipah, SARS-CoV-2, and chikungunya have been the cause of a significant rise in outbreaks and pandemics in India in recent years. Time-tested strategies for reducing the adverse consequences of these diseases continue to include early detection, reporting, and prompt public health response. The use of a trained Rapid Response Team to identify and address outbreaks in their early stages plays a crucial role in containing the spread of the disease.

6.2 Summary of the literature

- Epidemic intelligence—Europe

  All activities pertaining to the early detection of possible health risks, their validation, evaluation, and inquiry in order to suggest public health management measures are included in the field of epidemiological intelligence (EI). Both an indicator-based and an event-based component are integrated into EI. The term "indicator-based component" describes organized data gathered by standard surveillance systems. The term "event-based component" describes unstructured information obtained from any kind of intelligence source [9].

- One Health approach (developing One Health surveillance systems)

  The traditional approach to disease surveillance has been sector-specific, with distinct systems for monitoring the health of people, domestic animals, plants, wildlife, and the environment. In order to enhance prevention and mitigation of spillover events, One Health surveillance should incorporate integrated surveillance for both known and undiscovered pathogens. Additionally, in addition to this more conventional disease-based surveillance, it must incorporate surveillance of the factors that contribute to the onset of diseases [10].

  There is a National Joint Outbreak Response Team (NJORT) at the center. Further, as per the DO letter from JS (PH), MoHFW GOI, it was envisaged that State and District Surveillance Committees are to be constituted in all states/UTs. A similar surveillance committee may be formed at the corporation level, and accordingly, the same to be involved for outbreak response [11].

- Surveillance of ambulance dispatch data as a tool for early warning—Denmark

  Study conducted by the National Centre for Biological Defense, Statens Serum Institute, Copenhagen, Denmark. Ambulance dispatch data was collected. Data contained selected patient symptoms, patient characteristics, and geographical information. Subsequently, the data were spiked with epidemiological symptom data before analysis in order to simulate a geographically located, symptom-specific disease outbreak.

  An increased number of patients, for whatever reason, will, to a variable degree, influence transport statistics as well as other parameters, such as physician calls and emergency center statistics. Outcome—reducing the median outbreak detection time (MOD-Time) [12].

- Community-based surveillance

  Community-based surveillance may improve early detection and response to disease outbreaks by leveraging the capacity of community members to carry out surveillance activities within their communities.

- For the surveillance unit focusing on the schools, educational institutions, companies, etc., to report.

6.3 Key highlights and strategic recommendations

Surveillance units are envisioned with a system of the Health Emergency Operation Centre with trained human resources. A multidisciplinary team, including a public health specialist, microbiologist, and veterinarian, may be trained to detect any outbreak using various indicator-based and event-based early-warning signs through a One Health approach. Further encourage community members to report unusual events through the IHIP community-based reporting system. The aim is to have an outbreak detection and response mechanism through the surveillance unit.

7. Strengthening syndromic surveillance

7.1 Brief background of the topic

Emerging diseases may not fit into disease-specific definitions. Early detection of clusters of syndromes may trigger an alert before cases appear in a traditional surveillance system. In contrast to waiting for confirmed diagnoses, which can take longer to report, syndromic surveillance enables a quicker public health response by monitoring nonspecific symptoms and health-related behaviors in real-time, thereby providing an early-warning system to investigate and contain potential outbreaks before they become widespread. This makes syndromic surveillance crucial.

7.2 Summary of the literature

7.2.1 Syndromic surveillance in public health practice, New York City

The New York City Department of Health and Mental Hygiene has established a syndromic surveillance system that monitors emergency department visits to detect disease outbreaks early. Routinely collected chief complaint information is transmitted electronically to the health department daily and analyzed for temporal and spatial aberrations. Respiratory issues, fever, diarrhea, and vomiting are the key syndromes analyzed [13].

7.2.1.1 Participatory surveillance systems for ILI

Participatory surveillance systems for influenza-like illness (ILI) have proven to be accurate and reliable, with the detected timing and relative intensities of influenza epidemics being consistent with those reported by sentinel surveillance systems.

Influenzanet in Europe: Influenzanet is a participatory surveillance system monitoring the incidence of influenza-like illness (ILI) in Europe since 2003. It is based on data provided by volunteers who self-report their symptoms *via* the Internet throughout the influenza season and currently involves 10 countries [14].

FluTracking in Australia and New Zealand: FluTracking started with 400 participants in 2006 and now has more than 150,000 participants across Australia and New Zealand—making it one of the largest crowd-sourced public health surveillance systems in the world. More than 23,000 new "flutrackers" signed up in April 2020 alone, and that number is expected to grow as new clusters emerge [15].

In March 2020, health authorities in the United States (including the National Institute of Allergy and Infectious Diseases director Anthony Fauci) issued guidelines for American homes, schools, and workplaces.

WHO Report on 5 July 2024: Best practices for the design, implementation, analysis, and reporting of participatory surveillance for influenza-like illness [16].

Participatory surveillance for ILI is intended to complement traditional influenza surveillance and is not intended to function as event-based surveillance.

Similar reporting can be done in schools, apartment complexes, etc., in urban areas.

Syndromic surveillance systems for mass gatherings: Syndromic surveillance strategies have been utilized in a wide variety of mass gathering settings, including the London 2012 Olympic and Paralympic Games, the 8th Micronesian Games in 2014, and large camping events held by youth organizations. Syndromic surveillance at mass gatherings can be undertaken by the surveillance unit utilizing the Integrated Health Information Platform (IHIP) [17].

8. Entomological survey

8.1 Understanding the scope of entomology in disease control

The field of entomological surveillance entails covering all activities, procedures, and processes that are involved in the monitoring and management of vector-borne diseases in the specified area. The scope of these activities extends over aspects of transmission, detection, identification, and response to disease. The integrated entomological laboratory-based surveillance for vector-borne diseases such as malaria, chikungunya, dengue, Zika, leishmaniasis, lymphatic filariasis, and West Nile virus, including many other diseases, focuses on multiple vectors involved in disease vectoring, for example, mosquitoes and ticks. This includes monitoring the population dynamics, distribution, and behaviors of the vectors.

Vector-borne diseases, especially malaria and dengue, persistently rank as some of the most serious public health challenges across the globe. In India, malaria elimination is being pursued nationally with phased targets to achieve zero indigenous cases by 2027 and sustained elimination by 2030. Malaria claimed over 608,000 lives globally in 2022, and India accounts for a substantial burden in endemic regions. The main vectors of public health importance in India, such as *Anopheles, Aedes aegypti,* and *Aedes albopictus*, display different behaviors with widespread insecticide resistance. The most known symptomatic disease that affects humans, arboviruses, has more than 390 million infections worldwide each year. In India, based on epidemiological reports, dengue outbreaks are largely attributed to Aedes aegypti and Aedes albopictus. Therefore, strong entomological surveillance and an integrated vector management strategy are needed.

Even with all these advances in control strategies, such as insecticide-treated nets (ITNs), indoor residual spraying (IRS), and larval source management (LSM), mosquitoes are resisting insecticides and adapting their behavioral patterns for survival, so novel approaches are still needed. Novel methods like molecular surveillance and community-based interventions may help solve these problems.

A study in Benguela Province, Angola, highlighted the molecular characteristics of malaria vectors. Over 2200 adult mosquitoes were collected, with 733 identified as *Anopheles* species. Molecular analysis revealed a diverse vector population, including *Anopheles coluzzii*, *An. gambiae sensu stricto*, *An. arabiensis*, and *An. funestus*. Notably, *An. coluzzii*/*An. gambiae* hybrids were detected for the first time in this region.

Plasmodium falciparum infection rates varied significantly between urban (23.1%) and rural (5.7%) areas. Furthermore, knockdown resistance (kdr) mutations—L1014F and L1014S—were detected, underscoring the growing challenge of insecticide resistance. These findings call for continuous monitoring and tailored vector control strategies to mitigate malaria transmission in Angola [18].

Studies carried out in Rio Grande do Norte state, Brazil, have shown the value of virology in entomological surveillance. Out of the 1333 immature Aedes mosquitoes surveyed, Aedes aegypti accounted for 89% of the total. Molecular testing has shown very high rates of dengue virus (DENV) infection, with a 20.7% positive rate for pools of mosquitoes collected. The predominant serotype was found to be DENV-4, which was detected in 88.8% of the positive pools.

The minimum infection rate (MIR) for *Aedes aegypti* was 3.37, indicating a dire need for early-warning systems. This study has established that the detection of natural infections in mosquito populations would alert agencies to an impending outbreak, thus enabling them to take preemptive control measures on the vectors [19].

In Kampong Cham Province, Cambodia, a cluster-randomized trial assessed the impact of community-driven interventions on dengue vector populations. These interventions included the use of larvivorous guppy fish, mosquito traps, solid waste management, and behavioral education campaigns. Quantitative results demonstrated a 50% reduction in the Container Index (CI), a 45% reduction in the House Index (HI), and a 60% reduction in the Adult Index (AI) in the intervention areas, all statistically significant ($p < 0.002$).

While the results are promising, the study highlighted challenges in sustaining long-term impacts and translating entomological reductions into decreased dengue incidence. Community engagement and consistent follow-ups are crucial for maintaining these gains [20].

India's phased malaria elimination strategy has demonstrated significant progress, achieving a 27% reduction in malaria cases between 2017 and 2022. Entomological surveillance, supported by 103 zones, has been pivotal in monitoring vector species, their distribution, and resistance patterns. Interventions such as IRS and long lasting impregnated. Bednets (LLINs) have shown over 50% efficacy in reducing indoor vector density, while larval source management (LSM) has contributed to a 40% decline in mosquito breeding habitats in urban areas. These successes underscore the critical role of data-driven and integrated approaches in achieving elimination goals.

Resistance monitoring revealed widespread multi-insecticide resistance in *An. culicifacies*, a primary malaria vector. The integration of entomological and epidemiological data enables tailored interventions, particularly in high-transmission areas.

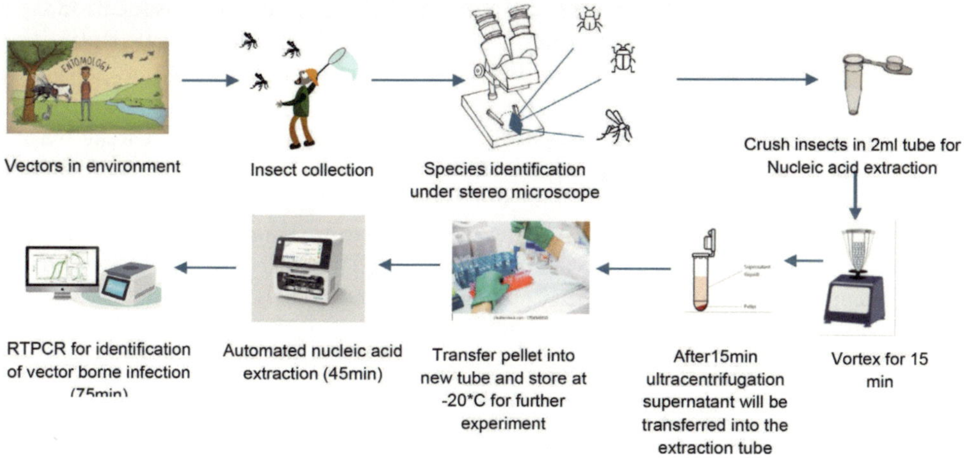

Figure 4.
Entomological molecular surveillance: Innovative VBD control strategy.

This model highlights the importance of scaling surveillance efforts to align with elimination goals (**Figure 4**) [21].

8.2 Strategic recommendations

1. Enhance molecular surveillance for data-driven decisions

   Quantitative molecular tools, such as PCR-based assays for kdr mutations and virological tests for pathogen detection, should be integrated into routine surveillance programs. In the Indian context, monitoring efforts have demonstrated that infection rates of *Plasmodium falciparum* declined by 27% between 2017 and 2022 due to targeted interventions. Additionally, integrated vector management strategies, including larval source management and the use of LLINs, have shown a reduction of mosquito breeding sites by 40% in urban regions. These metrics underline the critical importance of molecular tools and robust data collection for informing interventions.

2. Implement multipronged control strategies

   Vector control programs must adopt a holistic approach, combining larval source management, insecticide-based adult control, and community engagement. Successful examples include:

   - Cambodia: The use of guppy fish and solid waste management reduced entomological indices. Similarly, India's national vector borne disease control program (NNBDCP) program has successfully implemented larval source management (LSM) and insecticide-based strategies in select urban centers. However, the program's reach has been limited, with many cities yet to benefit from these interventions, highlighting the need for expanded implementation. The acceptance of such techniques within communities has been observed to be high, particularly when supported by educational campaigns and local engagement, offering an opportunity to scale these efforts nationwide.

- Brazil: Virological monitoring of *Aedes aegypti* provided early outbreak warnings. In India, under the nongovernmental organization initiative, a pilot was conducted at SCB Medical College, Cuttack, during the training of district microbiologists. This initiative successfully demonstrated the integration of entomological surveillance into existing health programs, gaining significant acceptance among community stakeholders and healthcare workers.

3. Strengthen early-warning systems

   Real-time surveillance data should be used to develop early-warning systems for outbreaks. For example, integrating entomological and virological data, as demonstrated in Brazil, can help identify hotspots and deploy resources effectively.

4. Address insecticide resistance

   Resistance management should be a priority. Regular monitoring of kdr mutations and other resistance mechanisms can guide the selection of effective insecticides. Diversifying control tools to include biological methods, such as larvivorous fish and microbial larvicides, can reduce reliance on chemical insecticides.

5. Foster community participation

   Community-driven initiatives are crucial for sustainable vector control. Educational campaigns targeting schools and local leaders can promote behavioral changes, such as the proper use of LLINs and the elimination of breeding sites.

   This has shown the potential of integrating molecular surveillance, community existence intervention, or adaptive management in a sound approach to vector-borne disease control. Such studies reviewed here have reported that such localized, context-specific, data-centered approaches need to be adapted specifically to the particular ecological and socio-cultural situations. By using molecular tools and building community involvement, we can further enhance the speed at which progress can be made toward malaria elimination and global dengue burden reduction.

9. Urban slum surveillance

Disease surveillance in urban slums: The challenges are manifold. One of the reasons is that even if these populations are recognized as part of a formal health system, many slum populations may still be excluded due to their informal living arrangements, lack of eligibility for legal recognition, and high mobility. A study conducted in one of the largest slums in Bangalore, Devarajeevanahalli, found that more than 40% of infectious disease cases are unreported due to small sample surveys and hospital reports [22]. Underreporting cases complicates the effective surveillance of disease trends and the introduction of timely preventive measures. In the same line, 30% of the diseases are not seen because of fragmented use by public and private health institutions in Mumbai. Such a scenario leaves wide gaps in data collection [23].

In addition, this arrangement has been worsened by the unavailability of well-structured, technology-enabled surveillance systems, which have allowed outbreaks that would have been detected to go unnoticed until they become serious public health problems. Even so, hope exists. The THULSI toolkit in Bangalore is a prime example of how real-time collection of data can serve as a breakthrough in disease detection. Using mobile technology, this intervention improved detection rates by over 20% and has therefore pointed the way for scalable, localized health technologies [22]. However, such tools remain out of reach for many urban slum communities, delaying responses to preventable outbreaks.

Fragmented healthcare access is making the problem worse. Slum residents use bits and pieces of public and private healthcare systems for their survival. They based the choice of a provider mainly on price and distance, rather than on how complete the system is. More than 60% of slum dwellers would rather use private providers, according to a study conducted in Mumbai. However, these private providers are hardly connected to an integrated surveillance mechanism. This leads to the unsuccessful integration of arising health threats into a good track and response action [23].

Environmental factors facilitating the spread of diseases in slums. A reduction in waterborne diseases of about 50% was recorded in Ahmedabad due to slum upgrading efforts, such as household water connections and sewage systems within those communities [24]. Over 40% of the denizens of Mumbai's underdeveloped slums suffer from recurrent bouts of waterborne diseases due to poor infrastructure [23]. These disparities highlight the direct relationship between environmental conditions and disease prevalence.

Local health facilities like Mohalla Clinics in Delhi, in some measure, would meet the health requirements of an underserved population but are faced with considerable limitations. Drug shortages, poor infrastructure, and a lack of awareness about the services hinder performance. Mohalla Clinics still hold promise for developing accessible health care based on further integrating stronger surveillance mechanisms [25].

9.1 Strategic recommendations for strengthening surveillance

1. *Develop integrated data systems*: Integrated health information systems are essential to bridge data gaps and enhance disease tracking. The integration of the THULSI toolkit with India's Integrated Health Information Platform (IHIP) could create a seamless system for digitizing health records and enabling real-time data collection. Community health workers can use the IHIP platform to report infectious diseases in real time, ensuring that local-level data from slum areas is synchronized with national health databases. This integration would significantly improve outbreak monitoring, early detection, and resource allocation [22].

2. *Implement community-based sentinel surveillance*: Community health officers (CHOs) can serve as the backbone of localized surveillance. Involving CHOs in Mumbai slums increased early detection of maternal and noncommunicable diseases by 30% [23]. Training CHOs to monitor disease trends and report cases using platforms like IHIP can ensure timely interventions and foster trust within the community.

3. *Enhance surveillance infrastructure*: Investments in technology-driven tools, such as electronic health records (EHRs) and GIS mapping, can significantly enhance surveillance capabilities. For instance, Mohalla Clinics in Delhi have piloted digital patient records to track disease prevalence effectively, providing a scalable model for other urban slums [25].

4. *Promote health education and awareness*: Health education campaigns tailored to local contexts can address misconceptions and improve participation in surveillance programs. In Bangalore, engaging community leaders and influencers increased participation in health screenings and treatment adherence [22]. Awareness initiatives should emphasize preventive measures such as vaccination and proper hygiene practices.

5. *Deploy mobile clinics and diagnostic tools*: Mobile health units equipped with point-of-care diagnostics bring healthcare directly to underserved populations. Delhi's Mohalla Clinics have demonstrated how proximity and affordability drive service utilization [25]. These mobile clinics can also serve as hubs for data collection, feeding valuable information into centralized surveillance systems.

10. Private sector involvement

The disease surveillance depends on the data reported from both the government and private health facilities. The National Family Health Survey (NFHS) highlighted that private health facilities serve a large portion of the population and handle a significant share of the disease burden. Thus, to capture the real disease burden and monitor the trends of a disease condition, the reporting from the private sector is equally crucial. It is envisioned to have a unified portal with a collaboration of both the public and private sectors for effective surveillance and public health action.

Use of digital health technologies: The adoption of digital platforms facilitates real-time data sharing between private health providers and IHIP. Mobile applications and electronic health records (EHRs) are critical for streamlining disease notification processes. The Kenya Health Information Systems Interoperability Framework (KHISIF) is an example of facilitating the interoperability of health information systems.

Policy and regulation: Policies promoting private sector involvement in surveillance can significantly improve reporting. For instance, the WHO's Global Framework for Private Sector Engagement in Health emphasizes creating regulatory environments that mandate disease reporting by private entities.

Legal and regulatory frameworks: Legislation mandating private sector reporting of notifiable diseases ensures compliance and accountability. The Public Health Act in countries like South Africa and Singapore includes provisions for private sector participation in disease surveillance.

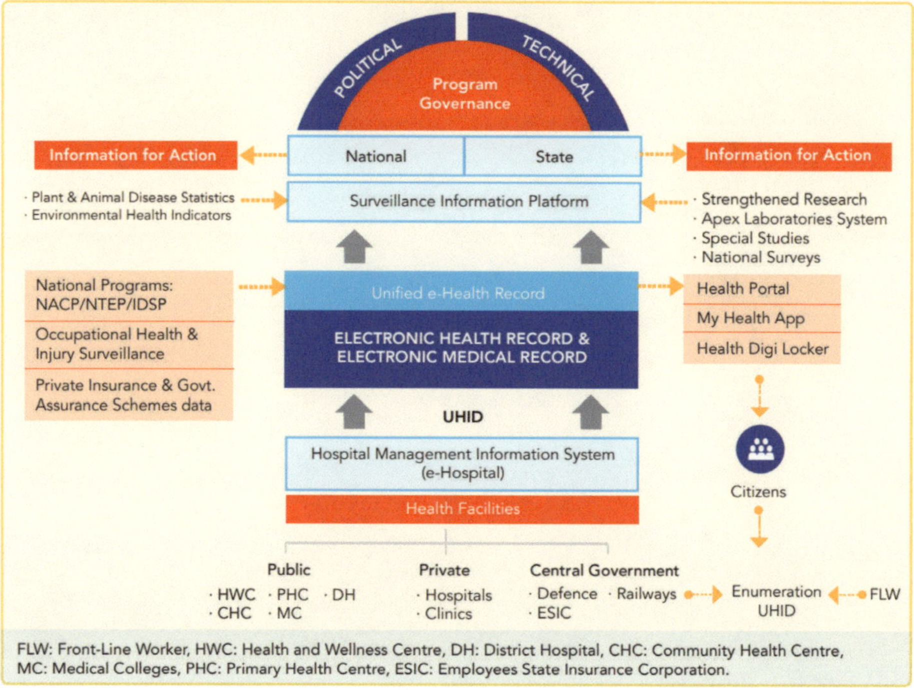

Figure 5.
*The architecture of public health surveillance in 2035 (*Courtesy: Vision 2035 NITI Ayog guideline*).*

Private Sector Engagement for Infectious Disease Surveillance in Mixed Health Systems: Lessons from a Model Dengue Reporting Network in India [26]. Developed and set up a public-private network (CODREN—Community Disease Detection and Response Network) with recruitment of eligible health resources (n = 462) in a municipal ward of Pune city.

It concluded that private sector engagement can improve dengue case detection with the selective inclusion of providers, sustained contact, feedback, and simple reporting methods.

NITI Aayog has highlighted the importance of private sector involvement in Disease Surveillance: Engaging the Private Sector.

Vision 2035 by NITI Aayog highlights the framework of the public health surveillance (**Figure 5**).

Private sector reporting from the private sector—Mangaluru, Karnataka:

> *Best practice—use of technology to better capture data on malaria cases from both the public and private sectors and impact on the malaria burden. The new "Malaria Control System" (MCS) was launched in October 2015 in Mangaluru by the Government of Karnataka to capture data and build the capacity of the existing program within the entire city. MCS was introduced as a program management system to support effective management of the malaria control program by digitizing reporting of newly diagnosed malaria cases for treatment, tracking, and closure of cases after completed care for each malaria patient.*

Author details

Danish Nasar Khan[1*] and Aliya Rizvi[2]

1 Program Management Unit for Health System Strengthening, Medhaj Techno Concept PVT, LTD, Lucknow, Uttar Pradesh, India

2 King George's Medical University, Lucknow, India

*Address all correspondence to: danishghazipur@gmail.com

References

[1] Jian SW, Chen CM, Lee CY, Liu DP. Real-time surveillance of infectious diseases: Taiwan's experience. Health Security. 2017;**15**(2):144-153. DOI: 10.1089/hs.2016.0107

[2] CDC. National Wastewater Surveillance System. Centers for Disease Control and Prevention. 2024. Available from: https://www.cdc.gov/nwss/index.html

[3] Anderson R et al. Simultaneous detection of SARS-CoV-2, influenza a, RSV, and measles in wastewater by multiplex RT-qPCR. Journal of Public Health Research. 2024;**33**(5):45-58

[4] Kim NY, Shi HJ, Oh SS, Gong YW, Kwon MJ, Eom JS, et al. Wastewater knows pathogen spread: Analysis of residential wastewater for infectious microorganisms including SARS-CoV-2. Infection and Chemotherapy. 2023;**55**(2):214-225. DOI: 10.3947/ic.2022.0152

[5] Mtetwa HN, Amoah ID, Kumari S, Bux F, Reddy P. Exploring the role of wastewater-based epidemiology in understanding tuberculosis burdens in Africa. The Lancet Global Health. 2023;**12**(7):672-685

[6] Chatterji A. Air Pollution in Delhi: Filling the Policy Gaps. Observer Research Foundation; 2020. Available from: https://www.orfonline.org/research/air-pollution-in-delhi-filling-the-policy-gaps

[7] Carver S et al. Environmental monitoring for infectious disease control. Journal of Environmental Monitoring. 2010;**12**:2048-2055

[8] Browne K, Mitchell BG. Multimodal environmental cleaning strategies to prevent healthcare-associated infections. Antimicrobial Resistance and Infection Control. 2023;**12**:83 DOI: 10.1186/s13756-023-01274-4

[9] Paquet C, Coulombier D, Kaiser R, Ciotti M. Epidemic intelligence: A new framework for strengthening disease surveillance in Europe. Euro Surveillance. 2006;**11**(12):pii=665

[10] Hayman TS, Adisasmito WB, Almuhairi S, Behravesh CB, Bilivogui P, Bukachi SA, et al. Developing one health surveillance systems. One Health. 2023;**17**:100617

[11] D.O letter of IDSP. Available from: https://idsp.mohfw.gov.in/showfile.php?lid=4301

[12] Bork KH, Klein BM, Mølbak K, Trautner S, Pedersen UB, Heegaard E. Surveillance of ambulance dispatch data as a tool for early warning. Euro Surveillance. 2006;**11**(12):pii=669

[13] Heffernan R, Mostashari F, Das D, Karpati A, Kulldorff M, Weiss D. Syndromic surveillance in public health practice, New York City. Emerging Infectious Diseases. 2004;**10**(5):858-864. DOI: 10.3201/eid1005.030646. Erratum in: Emerg Infect Dis. 2006;12(9):1472.

[14] Koppeschaar CE, Colizza V, Guerrisi C, Turbelin C, Duggan J, Edmunds WJ, et al. Influenzanet: Citizens among 10 countries collaborating to monitor influenza in Europe. JMIR Public Health and Surveillance. 2017;**3**(3):e66. DOI: 10.2196/publichealth.7429

[15] The University of Newcastle. Impact Case Study: FluTracking Update.

2020. Available from: https://www.newcastle.edu.au/__data/assets/pdf_file/0017/533420/UON-Impact-Case-Study-FluTracking-Update-August-2020.pdf

[16] World Health Organization. Best Practices for the Design, Implementation, Reporting and Analysis of Participatory Surveillance for Influenza-like Illness. 2024. Available from: https://www.who.int/publications/i/item/9789240095038

[17] Spector E, Zhang Y, Guo Y, Bost S, Yang X, Prosperi M, et al. Syndromic surveillance systems for mass gatherings: A scoping review. International Journal of Environmental Research and Public Health. 2022;**19**(8):4673. DOI: 10.3390/ijerph19084673

[18] Alves G, Troco AD, Seixas G, Pabst R, Francisco A, Pedro C, et al. Molecular and entomological surveillance of malaria vectors in urban and rural communities of Benguela Province, Angola. Parasites and Vectors. 2024;**17**:112. DOI: 10.1186/s13071-024-06214-8

[19] Medeiros AS, Costa DMP, Branco MSD, Sousa DMC, Monteiro JD, Galvão SPM, et al. Dengue virus in *Aedes aegypti* and *Aedes albopictus* in urban areas in the state of Rio Grande do Norte, Brazil: Importance of virological and entomological surveillance. PLoS One. 2018;**13**(3):e0194108. DOI: 10.1371/journal.pone.0194108

[20] Bigio J, Braack L, Chea T, Set S, Suon S, Echaubard P, et al. Entomological outcomes of cluster-randomised, community-driven dengue vector-suppression interventions in Kampong Cham province, Cambodia. PLoS Neglected Tropical Diseases. 2022;**16**(1):e0010028. DOI: 10.1371/journal.pntd.0010028

[21] Sharma RS, Sharma SN, Srivastava PK. Entomological surveillance and vector management towards malaria elimination in India. Journal of Communicable Diseases. 2023;**55**(1):35-39. DOI: 10.24321/0019.5138.202334

[22] George et al. Health issues in a Bangalore slum: Findings from a household survey using a mobile screening toolkit. BMC Public Health. 2019;**19**:456

[23] Naydenova E, Raghu A, Ernst J, et al. Healthcare choices in Mumbai slums: A cross-sectional study. Wellcome Open Research. 2018;**2**:115

[24] Butala et al. Improved health outcomes in urban slums through infrastructure upgrading. Social Science and Medicine. 2010;**71**:935-940

[25] Vohra RC et al. A study on the availability and accessibility of healthcare services provided at Mohalla clinics by the slum residents of Delhi. International Journal of Community Medicine and Public Health. 2022;**9**(6):2501-2507

[26] Furtado KM, Kar A. Private sector engagement for infectious disease surveillance in mixed health systems: Lessons from a model dengue reporting network in India. Journal of Health Management. 2022;**24**(4):583-592. DOI: 10.1177/09720634221091011

Chapter 6

Perspective Chapter: Clinical Impacts of Mpox Infection in Immunocompromised Patients

Maneesh Kumar, Pratima Gupta, Suman Kumar, Mithilesh Kumar Jha and Ratnesh Kumar

Abstract

In immunocompromised individuals, including HIV/AIDS patients, cancer patients, and those under post-transplant immunosuppression, Mpox infection is characteristically very severe and carries multiple complications. This study looks into the complexity of the clinical course of Mpox in these risk groups. The immunosuppressed present in most circumstances with severe skin lesions, unusual distribution of lesions, delayed wound healing, and visceral involvement. Complications like hemorrhagic Mpox, pneumonitis, encephalitis, persistent viremia, and persisting viral shedding increase the death risk manifold. Hemorrhagic and systemic clinical manifestations are most severe in cases with less than 200 CD4+ T-cells/μL. Besides, atypical presentations result in delayed diagnosis, which enhances transmission while complicating treatment. Also, there is a problem when it becomes chronic because of possible secondary infections, including bacterial and fungal superinfections. Improving outcomes is vital if this is diagnosed and treated promptly with polymerase chain reaction (PCR), cytokine profiling, and antiviral therapy (e.g., tecovirimat). Such ongoing infections commonly found within immunocompromised patients lead to viral escalation and prolonged hospitalization as well. Public health interventions ought to be made sophisticated and included in vaccination initiatives, educating patients, and controlling infections for those at high risk, particularly among the men who have sex with men and immunodeficiency disease population. This particular study highlights the urgent need for proposed clinical measures and global health initiatives aimed at the reduction of impacts caused by Mpox among the immunocompromised.

Keywords: HIV/AIDS, Mpox, hemorrhagic Mpox, immunocompromised patients, tecovirimat

1. Introduction

Mpox, formerly called monkeypox, is now a leading global health challenge and has proven detrimental to the health of particularly immunocompromised patients. The immunodeficient, for example, human immunodeficiency virus/Acquired immunodeficiency syndrome (HIV/AIDS), cancers, organ transplants, and individuals under immunosuppressive therapy, present particular clinical problems when infected with Mpox [1, 2]. While having a powerfully intact immune function, the differences arise when compared with an immunocompromised patient – infected persons are more prone to develop infections because of impaired surveillance functions [3, 4]. The gravity of such a situation may potentiate the formation of an unusual, vicious pathological condition. Prolonged viral shedding is among the main concerns raised in this class of patients, thereby extending the period of infectivity and increasing the risk of transmission in healthcare and community settings [5, 6]. Unusual clinical presentations can also be seen among immunocompromised patients, complicating clinical diagnosis and delaying early intervention [7]. Early identification may not be simple because fever, lymphadenopathy, or even the distinguishing rash sometimes do not appear or change [8, 9]. More often, such clinical symptoms increase the risk for disseminated disease since the virus penetrates beyond the skin and causes multiple organ systems to present extreme severe complications, including pneumonitis, encephalitis, and sepsis. The necrotic and hemorrhagic extensive skin lesions are commonly found among the immunocompromised hosts and indicate the aggressive nature of the disease [5, 9, 10].

One of the other more significant issues is the possibility that this type of population group could have treatment-resistant infections. Such patients may be immunocompromised and may not respond well to conventional therapy [11]. They may need to take more aggressive or combination therapies for longer durations. Vaccination, however, cannot help break the outbreak pattern; it becomes a new area of conflict. Similarly, live attenuated vaccines may be contraindicated in an immunosuppressed person, elicit suboptimal responses, and raise questions regarding possible safety concerns limiting their protective efficacy [12, 13]. Alarmingly, the mortality rates for Mpox infections are higher in immunocompromised individuals than in the general population by several folds. Studies have shown an increased risk of fatal outcomes, almost always associated with advanced immunosuppression or with multiple comorbidities. Hence, there is a crying need for specific treatment regimens aimed at early diagnosis, individualized therapy, and close follow-up [14, 15]. By creating a standardized treatment pathway with a multidisciplinary approach, clinical outcomes for this high-risk, vulnerable patient population could be optimized, and risks might be diminished. Surveillance and screening programs for Mpox should also target immunocompromised individuals, such as those affected by HIV/AIDS or that undergoing cancer treatment [12, 16, 17]. Train healthcare providers to recognize atypical manifestations of Mpox in such patients; these may not be the same as those for immunocompetent individuals. Further research should be directed toward developing antiviral therapies and prophylactic measures explicitly aimed at immunocompromised populations to mitigate the risk for severe Mpox infections [18].

Emerging Mpox infection increasingly correlates with the spread of travel and zoonotic reservoirs linking immune-compromised populations worldwide; hence, such phenomena cultivate the urge to intensify research and develop public health interventions [19]. What would be essential is knowing special clinical considerations and making those into feasible, actionable interventions aimed at minimizing morbidity and mortality for these populations. Timely diagnosis and effective intervention could go a long way in managing the course of the disease and preventing severe manifestations and complications [8, 20]. This study becomes increasingly important, as nearly all reports published discuss Mpox infections predominantly affecting the general population, with scant detailed information about immunocompromised patients. Given the clinical peculiarities, increased illness severity, and increased mortality observed in this vulnerable group, there is a need for targeted research that would inform public health and revamp clinical and policy practice. In addition to this, there are increasing numbers of immunocompromised individuals worldwide among transplant recipients, survivors of cancer, and those who have received long-term therapies with immunosuppressants, warranting the urgent need to know the behavior of Mpox in these populations [21, 22]. The gradual evolution of the Mpox virus and new emerging viral strains are expected to have various effects on immunocompromised hosts and thus strengthen the need for continuous monitoring and periodic revision of management protocols. Identifying unique risk factors and optimizing treatment protocols would, therefore, mean exploring vaccination approaches further in this group and would equate to better management outcomes for the affected individuals. Upgrading diagnostics and solid implementation of infection control measures should also be paramount to outbreak containment and protecting high-risk patients [23]. This study will critically assess the clinical impact of Mpox in immunocompromised populations to fill significant gaps in the knowledge that directly translate into interventions that improve patient care, create guidelines, and shape future research efforts.

2. Clinical presentation and progression

Mpox infections greatly influence patient health status according to the patient's type and severity of clinical features. In severely immunocompromised patients, skin lesions may lead to superinfection and scarring. An atypical rash distribution may delay diagnosis and risk transmission. The hemorrhagic condition of Mpox affects life-threatening situations with generalized bleeding and multiorgan failure, thereby demanding urgent supportive management [24]. Where the virus causes persistent shedding in blood and long-term presence in the bloodstream, it predisposes an infection to a prolonged duration and causes dissemination throughout the entire body (**Table 1**). This condition usually necessitates more treatment along with isolation.

When the lesions remain too long, they become chronic ulcers, which may open the victim to insidious invasion by secondary bacterial infections. The virus can target crucial organs such as the lungs and brain, causing unusual and severe complications like dreadful, extreme encephalitis and sepsis [21, 25]. The best outcomes will result from very early detection and diagnosis of the disease and prompt initiation of antiviral therapy, wound care, and supportive management.

2.1 Severe cutaneous lesions and atypical rash distribution

Mpox infection often shows a more acute and unusual clinical course in immunocompromised individuals than in the general population. A distinctive feature in immunocompromised patients is that severe skin lesions may occur. The incubation period is 6–13 days and can extend to 21 days. Specifically, the average is shorter, at 8.5 days, in cases following sexual activity. The first signs include low-grade fever, headache, and rashes in limited areas. Coupled with a cough, these may include dyspnea, runny nose, mouth ulcers, sore throat, weight loss, abdominal pain, and diarrhea. The lesions of the mucosa could penetrate the rectal wall. Some 85% of those with skin lesions also had lymphadenopathy [26]. Infections may, however, be

Clinical Features	Health Effects	Symptoms	Preventive Measures and Treatment	Examples
Severe Cutaneous Lesions	Skin infections, scarring, and disfigurement risk	Large limbs, necrotic and painful ulcers	Early use of antivirals, care of wounds	Necrotic skin lesions needing debridement
Atypical Rash Distribution	Delayed diagnosis and increasing transmission	Lesions on mucosa, genitals, or localized areas	Clinician alertness and training	Genital lesions mimicking sexually transmitted infections
Hemorrhagic Mpox	High mortality and multiorgan failure	Widespread bleeding, hematuria, internal bleeding	Aggressive supportive care and antivirals	Hemorrhagic rash and pulmonary hemorrhage
Prolonged Viral Shedding	Extended infectivity and risk of spread	Persistent detection of virus post-recovery	They are kept isolated and given extended antiviral therapy	Positive viral PCR several weeks after symptom resolution
Persistent Viremia	Systemically, it is spreading and poor prognosis	Continuous presence of the virus in the blood stream	Continuous and intensive monitoring and supportive therapy for patients	Prolonged viremia on blood tests
Delayed Wound Healing	Chronicity in wound, secondary infections	Nonhealing ulcers with superinfection	Optimizing wound management and treatment with antibiotics	Chronic skin ulcers with bacterial colonization
Visceral Dissemination	Multiorgan failure, increased mortality	Pneumonitis, hepatitis, encephalitis, sepsis	Early intensive care unit (ICU) management and aggressive antiviral management	Mpox-related encephalitis or acute respiratory distress syndrome

Table 1.
Elaborating clinical features and health impact during Mpox infection.

asymptomatic. For the healthy, lesions will migrate from face to limbs, while atypical for the immunocompromised. Mpox infection proceeds through the incubation, prodromal, rash, and crusting stages. The world health organization (WHO) divides Mpox Virus infection into an early five-day phase of fever, headache, and lymphadenopathy, followed by skin rash. Secondary fever may indicate resurgence; however, this may not be seen in pediatric patients [7]. In intact immune systems, skin lesions are usually limited to self-limiting lesions, whereas in immunocompromised hosts, necrotic skin lesions are generally large, deep, and relatively persistent. These lesions are very painful due to their size, cause severe damage to the host's well-being, act as a hindrance to therapy due to secondary infections, and may leave scars and create disfigurement. However, the patients have different problems from an impaired immune response (the pathology). The course and recovery are different. In July of the year 2022, Mpox was proclaimed as a public health emergency for the COVID-19 pandemic by the WHO. There are numerous barriers to access to diagnosis, immunization, and treatment in low-income countries. At the same time, all other known features of Mpox have also been found in immunocompetent persons [27]. In HIV-infected individuals, the infection is more virulent and severe than in individuals with normal antibody production and Th1 response, as this is the true nature of the disease.

The centers for disease control and prevention (CDC)'s September 2022 recommendations focused on immunocompromised populations suffering from the most severe stages of Mpox disease, particularly HIV-immune patients. Most severe cases were reported in patients with HIV and a cluster of differentiation 4 (CD4) count below 200 cells/mL [1, 26].

2.2 Hemorrhagic Mpox

Hemorrhagic Mpox (HMpox) is a sporadic yet complex disease mainly affecting immunocompromised individuals. This extensive bleeder bleeds through the skin and mucous membranes, significantly increasing mortality risk [24]. These symptoms point toward an intense invasion of the virus along with a wholly dysregulated immune response, requiring aggressive supportive care. The aggressive form of this disease is relative to the classic vesiculopustular type [28]. The severe manifestation is ascribed to great vascular destruction through an unchecked viral replication and an immune system failure that expresses itself in petechiae, ecchymoses, mucosal bleeding, hematuria, gastrointestinal bleeding, and possibly fatal hemorrhages in critical organs such as the lungs and the brain [29, 30]. HMpox is rapid in progression and most often has high mortality if not treated through aggressive supportive management like hydration, transfusions, antiviral therapy, and close hemodynamic monitoring. There are the highest incidences of this complication among immunocompromised persons, including the ones with advanced HIV infection (CD4+ T-cell count below 200 cells/μL), patients undergoing chemotherapy, transplant recipients receiving immunosuppressants, and individuals having certain primary immunodeficiencies [24, 30]. This year's Mpox outbreak fundamentally changed the landscape of risk around the world; over 18,000 cases were reported in Europe alone. The patterns of spreading evolved into primarily infecting men who have sex with men (MSM) through close physical or sexual contact, without travel to endemic regions. Undiagnosed and uncontrolled HIV will now become part of the risk population because they could be greatly immunocompromised without their knowledge, putting them at risk for severe or hemorrhagic forms of the disease [31, 32]. The emergence of HMpox has sounded the alarm on the need for rapid diagnosis, increased clinical vigilance, and expedited access to antivirals such as tecovirimat. Equally important is the demand for proper supportive care to calm the storm of bleeding and other derangements. Public health strategies should be directed toward vaccination, educating high-risk groups, improving diagnostics, and developing healthcare infrastructure to manage and treat complications [33].

2.3 Prolonged viral shedding

The transmission threat has exacerbated the chance of virus mutations, as has the virulence and transmissibility, all due to prolonged shedding from infected individuals within the immunocompromised population [34]. It is imperative to take urgent intervention steps for managing Mpox among vulnerable communities and strictly implement infection control procedures in healthcare environments. As demonstrated by the fast dissemination of Mpox globally in 2022, all of this will tell us about how connected the world is and how quickly infectious diseases can get tagged with a label of worldwide concern. The outbreak should be a reminder that the time is now for strong global health surveillance systems and an internationally coordinated response to emerging infectious diseases [1, 35]. In contrast, the other cases outside Africa were mainly associated with the spread of international travel and the importation of infected animals. Declining immunity from vaccination for smallpox and this Mpox outbreak has greatly favored transmission [35]. Increased morbidity and mortality, generally not associated with immunocompetent Mpox infection, severely affect these susceptible subgroups: patients with immunodeficiency, the elderly, small children, pregnant women, and those with comorbidities such as diabetes mellitus [36, 37]. Unlike many other outbreaks, over 95% of suspected transmission events have historical ties to sexual activity [36, 38]. Furthermore, most of the infected humans, about 98%, are probably gay or bisexual men, and out of these men, 41% were co-infected with HIV. Thus, it is reasonable to inquire whether Mpox could evolve into an sexually transmitted infection (STI) or indicate particularly at-risk communities [39]. The clinical suspicion for Mpox arises mainly from observing lesions and lymphadenopathy; however, the confirmatory diagnosis requires polymerase chain reaction (PCR) testing. There are bright hopes along with immunization through vaccines, repurposed antiviral agents, and stringent measures against the infection to control the disease. Most of what is known about Mpox relies now on information collected in resource-poor settings in Africa and thus needs to be reassessed in light of the recent global pandemic. The health agencies must unite worldwide to develop a common, well-funded research agenda and containment strategy to address this emerging threat [40, 41].

2.4 Persistent viremia

Persistent viremia is when viruses are continuously present in the bloodstream and not within the expected timescale, and this is more common in individuals with immunocompromised status. This indicates continued viral replication, which correlates with adverse clinical outcomes, namely systemic involvement and diversely affected organs [42, 43]. While features of Mpox are well known in individuals with standard immune systems, significant challenges related to diagnosis, vaccination, and treatment remain for low-income countries. In addition, immunocompromised persons are at increased risk of exposure and even death because they fail to produce adequate protective immune responses [43]. Although the origin of MpoxV is still unknown, a primary suspect is rodents. Consuming a raw or undercooked form of this contaminated meat can lead to exposure. People living far from such areas, close to forested areas, could also be exposed to infected animals. Mpox can be contracted through direct or indirect contact with infected body fluids or lesion materials. Direct exposure could contact fomites, respiratory secretions, and skin-to-skin contact [42, 44]. Injury indirect exposure can occur from 6 feet with patients undergoing specific procedures that generate aerosols of secretions, lesions, or dry exudates. Also, during childbirth and placental transmission, this virus is transmitted. The virus replicates in the initial site of infection and is sighted by mononuclear phagocytic cells, which diffuse through the whole pathway before returning to the dermal layer [45]. Initial replication occurs at the site of infection, wherein the virus reaches nearby lymph nodes and spreads into the bloodstream after 10–14 days [46]. Although it does not mention the primary immunodeficiency, it includes other types of disease conditions under autoimmune disease with immunodeficiency. Both immunocompetent and immunocompromised individuals face significant health risks, such as former immunosuppressed patients and old and young people. Characterized by prolonged infection, in-host viral evolution, and mutated viruses, this is the most frequently described infection among immunocompromised patients. Protracted bacterial bronchitis is found chiefly in children. Other infections associated with the immunocompromised condition are supported by blood, lung, and central nervous system viral, bacterial, and fungal infections [35, 47]. Such an immunocompromised condition makes patients more prone to prolonged infections, increasing hospital stays and complications. Studies in response to infection of the immunosuppressed range in terms of mortality, complications, and the duration of hospital stay [42]. A study conducted in Spain in 2009 showed that immunocompromised individuals share a higher mortality rate than immunocompromised individuals with Influenza A (H1N1), and bacterial coinfections complicated many cases. However, a study in 2020 from the United States reported that long-term usage of immunosuppressive drugs was not associated with worse clinical outcomes for patients with COVID-19 hospitalized. Another study concluded that those immunosuppressed patients contracting COVID-19 did not have a higher chance of getting severe lung disease; therefore, treatment, including chemotherapy, can continue [48, 49]. There are controversies concerning immune suppression in pregnant females, where susceptibility to infections depends not only on the woman's immune status but also on the particular placental immune response to specific pathogens.

2.5 Delayed wound healing

Delayed wound healing constitutes a frequent and complex complication of Mpox infection, specifically a more significant challenge among the immunocompromised. This is purely because of the direct cytopathic effect of the virus on skin cells and the poor regenerative capacity of the host [50]. However, an immunocompetent person would usually experience complete healing of a cut in different stages and dry after a few weeks. This could take months for immunodeficient individuals or patients suffering from conditions like diabetes or HIV [51, 52]. Prolonged injury would leave these lesions open and ulcerated and remain inflamed for days, weeks, and even longer, leading to significant gaps in the skin barrier. Chronic ulcers can be a classic entry point for subsequent bacterial or fungal infections [53]. For example, some such superinfections would include those associated with *Staphylococcus aureus* or *Pseudomonas aeruginosa* infections in Mpox lesions that do not heal once untreated, causing agonizing pain, suppuration, cellulitis, or, in the extreme, systemic sepsis [54]. Chronic wounds may also become colonized by other pathogens, including species of *Candida,* to make matters worse. Again, in addition to the antiviral therapy, the treatment for these secondary infections must include specific antibiotic or antifungal therapy. It also causes extensive scarring, contractures, and disfigurements that endure long-term in the worst-affected cases. Thus, all good wound care, identification of superinfection, and combined therapy become very important in the healing process while minimizing complications and improving the patient's outcome [55, 56].

In their research conducted in 2024, Azzam et al. [57] present an insightful discussion of the effects of immunosuppression on the severity and mortality of Mpox, with an important consideration for visceral dissemination in the immunocompromised population. The visceral spread probably becomes a significant complication of Mpox infection only among individuals who happen to have an immune-weakening condition, such as those with very advanced HIV infections (CD4 counts of below 200 cells/μL) and organ transplant recipients. In post-mortem studies, testing by PCR and immunostaining has shown Mpox in various visceral locales, indicating it is truly systemically involved. Severe disease manifestations include respiratory failure, hepatitis, enterocolitis, encephalitis, and sepsis. In turn, these complicate the condition and increase the risk of death [56, 57]. The virus spreads through the bloodstream and lymphatic system, with help from leukocytes and lymph nodes, reaching distant organs. Immunocompromised patients, particularly those with uncontrolled HIV infection and low CD4 counts, have been found to present significantly high levels of viral dissemination [58]. This widespread spread of Mpox can probably cause multi-organ failure in the immunocompromised host. The virus infects different cell types and tissues; thus, it shows the importance of identification and early intervention to prevent severe complications. Mechanisms of viral spread and organ tropism become important for developing therapy capable of being applied to targeted therapy and improving outcomes with patients with severe Mpox presentations. In addition to the cytopathic effects of the virus, immune system dysregulation secondary to hemophagocytic lymphohistiocytosis (HLH) and immune reconstitution inflammatory syndrome (IRIS) can also attack and destroy tissue [57, 58]. Due to the cytokine storms that HLH would generate, it would cause multiorgan failure; IRIS would then complicate disease management in patients with HIV. Coinfection with bacteria, fungi, and viral pathogens contributed to poor treatment outcomes. Results indicate that these two mechanisms- visceral dissemination and immune system dysregulation- cause rapid clinical deterioration. Clinicians should maintain a high suspicion that visceral involvement exists in immunocompromised patients if severe symptoms arise. Diagnosis will be established through imaging, laboratory investigations, and tissue biopsy. The study highlights the pressing need for early diagnosis and monitoring and the initiation of antiviral therapy for all immunocompromised individuals to prevent the fatal consequences of visceral dissemination [24, 57].

3. Immunocompromised host factors

Mpox infection is a growing health problem, especially for people with weak immune systems. These people can get very sick because their bodies cannot fight infections well. Conditions like HIV/AIDS, cancer, or certain medicines can weaken the immune system [58]. These medicines are often used after organ transplants or during some treatments. When the immune system is weak, the Mpox virus can spread more easily and cause worse symptoms [59]. These patients might also have other infections at the same time, making it harder to diagnose and treat them. Some treatments and vaccines might not work well or could cause problems for them [27, 59]. So, it is important to spot symptoms early, use the right antiviral medicines, and carefully plan each patient's treatment [60]. Raising awareness and improving medical care for people with weak immune systems can help lower risks and improve outcomes for those with Mpox [28, 61].

3.1 HIV/AIDS-associated Mpox

In HIV/AIDS-related Mpox, the magnitude of the CD4+ T cell loss dramatically influences the level of susceptibility to infection. CD4+ T-cells are responsible for coordinating the adaptive immune response by activating destruction mechanisms *via* cytotoxic T-cells and macrophages in order to control viral infections. And when the CD4+ count drops to under a critical level of 200 cells/μL—that is, a clinical marker for advanced immunosuppression—the body's ability to resist the Mpox tends to be seriously impaired [62]. This defect in the immune system allows the virus to replicate unfettered, leading to an abrupt spread throughout the body. In the clinical setting, the late stage HIV-infected patients with low CD4+ + T-cells showed atypical Mpox and severe symptoms. These consist of severe mucocutaneous lesions, wound healing retardation, necrotic ulcerations, and systemic manifestations (pneumonitis, meningo-encephalitis, and prolonged viremia). Furthermore, the immunocompromised condition increases susceptibility to secondary infections such as those of bacterial, fungal, and other viral origins. These coinfections not only aggravate the clinical picture but also represent a potential cause of disruption from the diagnostic point of view and may hide the symptoms of Mpox and delay the appropriate therapy [58].

In addition to HIV/AIDS, other immunocompromised groups—chronic users of immunosuppressive therapy (e.g., corticosteroids and biologics), cancer chemotherapy patients, and organ transplant recipients—face similar risk. In such patients, chemotherapeutics compromise both innate and adaptive immune arms and compromise antiviral defenses, rendering an environment permissive for Mpox replication and advancement. Transplant recipients are specifically at increased risk due to lifelong maintenance of immunosuppression for prevention of graft rejection, resulting in a paradoxical vulnerability to infections such as Mpox. In addition, primary immunodeficiencies such as severe combined immunodeficiency (SCID) and common variable immunodeficiency (CVID) are inherited diseases in critical immune pathways. These individuals often have recurrent infections and inadequate vaccine responses and are significantly at risk for Mpox-related sequelae. This increased risk makes early diagnosis using PCR and cytokine profiling, early initiation of antiviral therapy such as tecovirimat, and close monitoring for complications, critical in the clinical management of Mpox especially in the immunocompromised, and in particular, individuals with HIV/AIDS and CD4 + T-cell depletion. Customized therapy, early detection, and promoting public health are key strategies for reducing the burden of cancer in these vulnerable populations [54, 61, 63].

3.2 CD4+ T-cell depletion

The mechanisms underlying and the severity of Mpox, especially among those most susceptible, involve CD4(+) T-cell depletion. During this disease, they are rapidly involved in boosting antiviral immunity through CD8+ T-cell-based mechanisms and supporting antiviral B-cell responses, and also directly, through secretion of antiviral cytokines such as interferon-gamma (IFN-γ) [64]. In advanced HIV/AIDS, the count falls below 200 cells/μL, and is a dangerous threshold below which the immune system loses its ability to combat life-threatening infections [65]. Previous studies have revealed that Av-specific Th1 effector memory CD4+ T cells are required and sufficient for the tissue prophylaxis of poxvirus infection, such as Mpox. These stratified, specialized memory T cells would be rapidly deposited at the site of infection, specifically the skin, and secrete IFN-γ upon antigen-specific stimulation [66]. But other primary skin cells would be enhanced for local antigen presentation, the establishment of an antiviral state, and IFN-γ effect on MHC class I and II expression on keratinocytes. In the absence of functional CD4+ T cells, these protective processes are ineffective, and the virus replicates unimpeded and spreads to other organs, including the lung, liver, intestine, and brain [67]. The immune control of these opportunistic organisms is also lost as a result of CD4+ T-cell depletion. Such disease predisposition particularly makes those with such profoundly weakened immunity highly susceptible to Mpox or even other secondary bacteriological/fungal, or viral coinfections, which complicates management and augments mortal risk. This also highlighted that this zoonotic pox is Mpox-i, that is, evolved strategies to

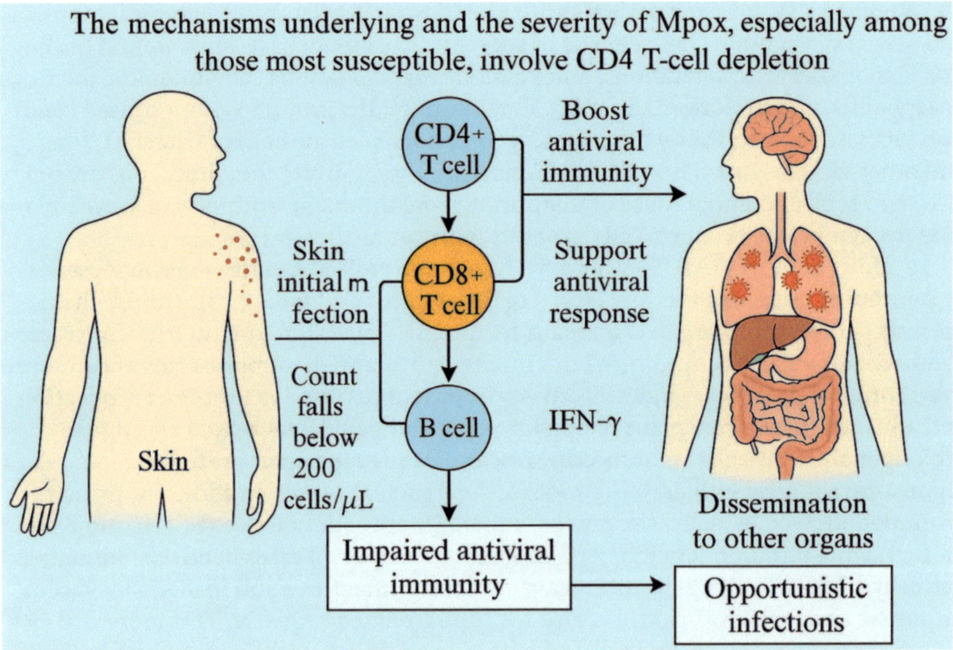

Figure 1.
CD4+ T-cell depletion that leads to ineffective antiviral immunity in a Mpox disease, evoking the viral transfer to other tissues and increasing the risk for opportunistic infections.

avoid detection by CD8+ T-cells by downregulation of MHC class I expression [68]. Hence, the host is rendered extremely susceptible as there are no functional CD4+ T cells to trigger compensatory immune responses from keratinocytes or other antigen-presenting cells. This needs to be considered not only concerning possible vaccination strategies in this context. Conventional live vaccinia virus vaccine induces excessive Th1 memory. However, newer non-replicating vaccines, such as modified vaccinia ankara (MVA), have failed to elicit such potent Th1 CD4+ T-cell responses and likely also leave this group of immunocompromised individuals less protected [69]. Monitoring of CD4+ T-cell counts, early antivirals, and a better vaccine formulation would not be overblown tactics in combating the effects of Mpox in this high-risk group specifically (**Figure 1**).

3.3 Opportunistic coinfections

The global outbreaks of Mpox during the 2022–2023 timeframe starkly pointed toward Mpox coinfection rates, highly pronounced among certain risk group members: MSM. Besides, the studies show that, on average, more than 35% of Mpox cases are reported in persons with HIV [70]. Also, over 40% have other STI infections, such as Chlamydia, Gonorrhea, Syphilis, and herpes, apart from infection by bacterial pathogens such as *Staphylococcus aureus* and Group A Streptococcus. These coinfections below add complexity and diversity to the clinical picture [7, 71]. First, HIV disrupts immune regulation, especially among those with low CD4+ T-cell counts, and limits the ability of the body to control the replication of Mpox, thus allowing more progression of the disease. A further complication arises from coinfection with herpes simplex virus (HSV-2), whereby genital lesions become more severe by attacking similar cell types, Langerhans cells, dendritic cells, and macrophages, already sickened by Mpox [72]. It allows viral entry into the circulation, compromises skin barriers, and facilitates systemic dissemination with subsequent visceral involvement. Similarly, superinfection with group a streptococcus (GAS) could predispose to an explosive inflammatory response with respiratory sequelae. GAS attaches to airway epithelial cells, invades them, kills them, and injures the underlying vascular structures. This damage clears the way for bacterial entry to the bloodstream, thus allowing entry for the Mpox virus and worsening the disease process within the body, as in sepsis. Infected tissue infiltrates macrophages and dendritic cells, yet in an immunocompromised host, these cells become infected by Mpox, thereby inducing more immunosuppressive effects [73]. Coinfections also complicate diagnosis. Clinical features that overlap, such as vesicular rashes from HSV or ulcerative lesions from syphilis, can mask Mpox infection and delay its diagnosis and management [74]. Molecular testing that detects orthopoxviruses but does not differentiate Mpox from other viruses, such as molluscum contagiosum virus (MOCV), gives erroneous results and complicates clinical decision-making. From a therapeutic point of view, opportunistic coinfections would reduce the efficacy of antiviral regimens like tecovirimat. According to some reports, coinfection with secondary syphilis delayed the Mpox clearance despite total antiviral treatment [75, 76]. Moreover, during ongoing infection, under antiviral pressure, substantially virus-resistant strains will be selected, especially for patients with uncontrolled HIV infection. There have been reports that advanced-stage HIV-infected individuals may have high resistance rates to tecovirimat (CD4+ T-cell count <35/μL) and the new treatment for syphilis [77]. Coinfection therapies are closely observed for potential interactions with Mpox medications. It is anticipated that tecovirimat will reduce serum-iripivirine levels and, due to a hypothesized increased concentration of brincidofovir, increase the toxicity of some agents, such as protease inhibitors. Thus, Mpox coinfections need more complex multidisciplinary management [78].

3.4 Immunosuppressive therapy

Given the fact that severe cases of Mpox infection have increased, immunosuppressive therapy is often given in cases of autoimmunity, cancers, and post-organ transplantations. Glucocorticoids, calcineurin inhibitors such as tacrolimus or cyclosporine, and various biological therapies targeting tumor necrosis factor (TNF) and interleukins interfere with innate and adaptive immune functions. Due to immunity suppression, extended viral replication occurs in these individuals, leading to poor viral clearance, prolonged shedding, and systemic dissemination of Mpox [79]. The CDC claims that patients with active immunosuppressive therapy usually present cases of severe Mpox with rash over large areas, necrotizing lesions, ocular involvement, pulmonary disorders, encephalitis, and septicemia [80]. In these instances, other microbial infections can be controlled due to a lack of immune surveillance. Bacterial coinfections with *Staphylococcus aureus* and *Streptococcus pyogenes*, fungal infections with Candida species, and viral infections, most especially cytomegalovirus (CMV), are frequently noted in these cases. The latter contributes to tissue destruction that impedes healing and dramatically increases the possibility of multiorgan failure [81]. T-cell and macrophage suppression due to therapy with corticosteroids or calcineurin inhibitors leads to failure of antiviral response, which is important in controlling Mpox. In this way, even locally invasive infections become quickly lethal. The presence of biologics targeting TNF or interleukins further hampers inflammatory responses necessary for viral containment. Likewise, in a similar continuum, the article further adds that Mpox confections with STIs are frequent among immunocompromised persons −41% of Mpox patients had an STI diagnosis during the last 12 months in the United States during the 2022 outbreak [68, 82]. STIs may create mucosal lesions when Mpox enters and is disseminated throughout the body. In contrast, skin lesions caused by Mpox may predispose an infected person to a secondary infection. Mpox is especially hard to manage in immunosuppressed patients. Antiviral treatment early in the disease course with tecovirimat may be advisable, but it would depend on careful evaluation of drug-drug interactions [58, 83]. Tecovirimat would lower serum levels of immunosuppressants, especially tacrolimus and sirolimus, thus requiring close therapeutic monitoring. If oral absorption is affected or the severity has been wrought, use intravenous tecovirimat, perhaps prolonged beyond 14 days, and other adjunctive therapies such as brincidofovir or cidofovir. Finally, the immunization approaches are also different for this population. The non-replicative Modified Vaccinia Ankara vaccine JYNNEOS is assumed to be safe in immunocompromised patients; however, the live replicating ACAM2000 vaccine is contraindicated due to the risk of serious complications related to vaccination [72, 84].

3.5 Cancer-related immunosuppression

The outbreaks of Mpox have introduced new public health problems afflicting different immunocompromised groups, particularly cancer patients. The research's purpose was to gauge understanding and lethargy toward the Mpox vaccine among cancer patients in light of increasing misinformation surrounding COVID-19. Their viewpoints would, therefore, weigh heavily on availing this particular group of immunocompromised patients, though their conditions and treatments put them at increased risk of severe Mpox infection. A cross-sectional survey among 275 cancer patients used structured questions to assess the sociodemographic background, knowledge about Mpox, attitudes toward vaccination, and intention to accept the Mpox vaccination [85]. Results were littered with significant knowledge gaps and a landscape showing vaccination hesitancy. While 73.1% could have desired more details about Mpox, only 33.8% trusted the global efforts controlling the outbreak [86]. Interestingly, 69.1% of patients remained skeptical about receiving the Mpox vaccine, primarily due to safety concerns and other interactions with ongoing cancer treatments. Further multivariate logistic regressions revealed essential predictors of the willingness to get vaccinated. Younger people, especially those younger than 65, were likely more receptive to new public health interventions. Besides, patients who had previously heard about Mpox and understood it somewhat were more inclined toward accepting the vaccine. It proves that correct information and education can significantly influence the health behavior of vulnerable populations. The study concludes that, in Turkey, many cancer patients remain reluctant to be vaccinated against Mpox despite increased susceptibility [85, 87]. They are among the strongest deterrents to safety and possible interaction with their cancer therapies. Critical to the immediate implementation of targeted education interventions that improve vaccine uptake in high-risk groups is such reassurance, priority given to educating the patients regarding potential risks that the vaccine might pose to cancer treatments, and clarification of how vaccination might fit into their cancer management protocols. Dialog grounded in well-understood evidence will be critical to instilling trust and knowledge in patients against this vulnerable population with threats emerging from infectious agents like Mpox [87].

3.6 Post-transplant recipients

Post-transplant individuals are most vulnerable to severe Mpox infections as a result of the long-term state of immunosuppression, which continues to prevent the rejection of the graft. Calcineurin inhibitors like tacrolimus, corticosteroids, and anti-proliferative agents like mycophenolate mofetil or azathioprine form the immunosuppressive regimens that are brought together to damage innate adaptive immunity [88]. Innate and adaptive immunity are highly impaired, with signs of diminished immune response resulting in fast replication of the Mpox virus, dissemination, and delayed clearance, leading to the disease becoming more aggressive and associated with increased morbidity [89]. Suliman et al. [90] provided data about Mpox cases through a study on kidney transplant recipients and identified several main clinical trends in reported cases. Of the 12 publications concerning case reports and series, most patients were male, with a median age of 43. The manifestations of these patients include widespread vesiculopapular or nodular rashes, mucosal ulcerations, systemic symptoms (fever, fatigue, diarrhea), and, in some cases, organ-specific complications such as pneumonitis, encephalopathy, and multiorgan failure [90]. For example, one patient experienced encephalopathy and multiorgan failure, eventually leading to death even with active care measures. In contrast, another patient died within 3 days of hospitalization due to pneumonitis with circulatory shock. A huge concern is delayed diagnosis among post-transplant patients, for the initial signs of fever and rash may be misinterpreted as initial signs associated with opportunistic infection or drug side effects. Early suspicion and intervention become increasingly mandatory because of this doubt and its potentially rapid course. Atypical rashes, mucosal ulcers, or unexplained systemic illnesses in transplant recipients should prompt Mpox consideration, especially if epidemiologically linked to known outbreaks. Most importantly, however, management strategies need to be tailored in detail. Most patients were treated with tecovirimat and supportive care, the first-line antiviral for Mpox [91, 92]. Aspirin may be helpful when renal immune recovery is needed by reducing calcineurin inhibitors or withholding antiproliferative agents. Some patients also completed treatment with brincidofovir (as an alternative antiviral) with no serious adverse events attributable to the drug. Lastly, antibiotics were used empirically as secondary bacterial infections with *Staphylococcus aureus, Pseudomonas aeruginosa*, and *Escherichia coli* further burdened the clinical course. While the majority of the reported patients did recover, there were considerable variations in the duration of illness, with some patients taking longer than 2 months for complete resolution of symptoms [92]. Furthermore, post-discharge respiratory complications were noted, demonstrating possible long-term sequelae for nonlethal cases. There are no allegations of acute kidney injury directly from Mpox. The present state of affairs, however, does leave an area of intense concern, that is, the complexity involved in managing renal function within a transplant recipient at risk for acute kidney injury resulting from other means apart from Mpox [93].

4. Complications and severity

With Mpox in immunocompromised persons, one of the major complications is severe lymphadenopathy, notably different from that seen in immunocompetent hosts. In otherwise healthy hosts, lymphadenopathy tends to be localized, somewhat uncomfortable, and self-limiting, with a duration of days to a week, while the immune system deals with viral replication [93]. Uncompromised patients, mainly those who are advanced HIV/AIDS, cancer, or on any type of immunosuppressive therapies, will have generalized, extremely painful lymph nodes for a much more extended period [94]. This would indicate an inappropriate response whereby the host body cannot mount a response to contain the Mpox virus, allowing it to replicate further and access the systemic compartment. Enlarged lymph nodes in the neck, axillary, or inguinal regions, or even within the abdominal cavity, can be clinically detected along with possible mild fever, fatigue, and pain during motion or even on palpation [24, 94]. Such a context involves a patient with poorly controlled HIV infection: a CD4+ T-cell count of less than 100 cells/μL presenting with painful bilateral inguinal lymphadenopathy and skin ulceration over the genital region. In some patients, necrotizing lymphadenitis occurs, wherein infected lymph nodes become necrotic, worsen the clinical picture, and complicate the course with bacterial superinfection. Persistent lymphadenopathy can also be a reservoir for persistent viral shedding, increasing infectivity and delaying recovery. CT or ultrasound imaging studies often demonstrate the presence of enlarged, inflamed, poorly demarcated lymph nodes, causing concern for coexisting bacterial or mycobacterial infections. In advanced cases, lymph node biopsy would help differentiate Mpox-associated lymphadenopathy from important malignancies, particularly lymphoma, which is very common in the immunocompromised population [95].

Neurological complications, while relatively uncommon in Mpox infection, remain a profound concern within the immunocompromised population, often culminating in grave outcomes. Those immune-compromised individuals in whom advanced HIV/AIDS or immunosuppressant therapy permits lower immune surveillance allow the virus into the central nervous system (CNS), leading to encephalitis or myelitis [96]. Encephalitis, or inflammation of the brain tissue itself, has been documented in cases of Mpox infection in patients with impaired immunity [97]. Neuroimaging showed evidence of diffuse brain inflammation. Cerebrospinal fluid (CSF) testing confirmed the presence of orthopoxvirus DNA. Long-term cognitive impairment was noted in the patient despite treatment with tecovirimat and intensive supportive care. It was managed through high-dose corticosteroids, empirical antimicrobial therapy, prolonged hospital stays, and partial neurological recovery. Hematogenous dissemination of the virus or infected monocytes and lymphocytes traversing the blood-brain barrier is the presumed mechanism of these events [98]. In an ordinary host, immune responses would have prevented this virus from entering the CNS. However, in the case of immunocompromised hosts, impaired response, reduced CD4+ T-cell, and cytotoxic T-cell response cannot check and control the viral replication, thus permitting viral dissemination to neurologically sensitive tissues. Depending on the degree of CNS involvement, the future course of Mpox-associated neurological features will identify cognitive impairment, motor dysfunction, epilepsy, and chronic neuropathic pain [3].

5. Diagnosis and biomarkers of Mpox in immunocompromised patients

Accurate and timely diagnosis of Mpox among immunocompromised individuals is the most crucial thing, since delayed detection might lead to rapid progressive disease, severely complicated conditions, and increased mortality. As the clinical picture is atypical and disease dissemination is possible, a comprehensive diagnosis is necessary: molecular, serologic, virologic, and pathologic tests. Detection of viral

Mpox DNA by polymerase chain reaction (PCR), commonly obtained from lesion smears, crusts, or exudates, forms the backbone of Mpox diagnosis [99, 100]. PCR remains the most sensitive and specific test available. This is even more imperative in immunocompromised patients with lesions that present as unusual, mucosal, or internal lesions with possibly minimal pustules and clinical challenges in identifying them. Alongside PCR for lesions, blood, cerebrospinal fluid, or other body fluids, tracing dissemination of the disease systemically can also be aided by serological testing by detection of immunoglobulin M or G antibodies; however, in retrospective studies or in cases where PCR results could not be obtained, this type of testing could play a role. Again, antibody response might be reduced or delayed in weak patients with compromised B-cell function, restricting serologic confirmation as a primary diagnostic tool in many instances [100, 101]. Nevertheless, when the absence of serologic response is analyzed in conjunction with a clinical index of suspicion, this may denote profound immunosuppression. Although not commonly performed in regular practice, viral load testing can have significant prognostic value in immunocompromised patients. Just as blood Mpox viral loads or lesion samples have been associated with severe disease and longer disease duration, a greater incidence of complications, including encephalitis, pneumonitis, and multisystem organ failure, is to be noted. Quantitative PCR, where applicable, can also be used to determine treatment effects, particularly in patients undergoing antiviral therapy with tecovirimat or cidofovir. Immune dysfunction under severe Mpox status mainly relates to markers of cytokine storm. In the serum of an immune-compromised host, cytokines such as interleukin 6 (IL-6), TNF-α, and IFN-γ are at an elevated level [102]. A rupture of tissues, causing multiple organ functions that will affect the clinical course, results from this hyperinflammatory response. The cytokine profile may hence be employed for stratification of patients into syndromes with different severities and for instituting adjunct therapy with immunomodulators or corticosteroids in select situations. Histopathological findings are relevant, especially in atypical or deeply seated Mpox cases. Skin or other organ biopsies may show classical findings like ballooning degeneration of keratinocytes, necrosis, vasculitis, and viral inclusion bodies. When PCR is inconclusive, immunohistochemistry and/or *in situ* hybridization can establish viral etiologies or differentiate those from other pathologies, disease reaction, herpes virus infection, or lymphoma.

6. Future prospects of Mpox in immunocompromised patients and its cure

In this dynamic landscape of global health, the growing burden of Mpox, particularly its severe impact on the immunocompromised, calls for the development of integrated and forward-looking strategies involving clinical and diagnostic studies as well as therapeutic and public health approaches. New epidemiology studies have revealed a characteristic clinical course of Mpox in many high-risk groups, such as patients with HIV/AIDS, patients with malignancies, transplant recipients, and patients treated with immunosuppressive regimens [103]. But as with all things, disease epidemiology is constantly changing, and management protocols need to continue to evolve and be refined. Novel diagnostic options will be key for early diagnosis and rational therapy selection. Innovative technologies include rapid molecular point-of-care PCR assays, viral load quantization, and multiplex molecular platforms with the ability to detect coinfections (bacterial, fungal, sexually transmitted) and are likely to improve diagnostic accuracy [104]. Cytokine profiling combined with immune biomarkers is also promising in predicting the severity of the disease as well as in guiding immunomodulatory interventions [105]. Transfer digital tools, for example, telepathology and AI-assisted histopathological interpretation, may increase the correctness and availability of diagnosis, especially in settings with few resources. From a clinical standpoint, studies need to explore which antiviral treatment can be optimally intensified, including both optimizing the dosing and duration of tecovirimat and considering whether combinations of antiviral therapy targeting the patterns of immunosuppression will be useful. Individual treatment approaches, which could be based on the patient's immune status and comorbidities or coinfection loads, will then be critical for enhancing the maximal effectiveness of the therapies [106, 107]. In addition, long-term follow-up studies are required to define and treat the outcomes of Mpox, especially its neurological and ophthalmological sequelae, and to establish postinfection monitoring and rehabilitation recommendations. There is a strong preventive rationale for the use of non-replicating vaccines such as JYNNEOS in the immunocompromised population. Advances in vaccine development should focus on enhancing immunogenicity without sacrificing the safety of the vaccine. Targeted educational efforts to address vaccine hesitancy, especially in patients with cancer and transplant recipients, are critical to increase coverage and ensure community immunity. In policy dimensions, investment in surveillance systems and promotion of real-time data sharing, as well as including immunocompromised individuals to be part of the target in clinical trials and vaccine registration roll-out, are important factors toward achieving equitable health care values. Global site and context-specific clinical guidelines for the management of Mpox in immunosuppressed persons will aid in standardization and quality of care in different settings. In the end, the vision for a future of Mpox management in immunocompromised hosts will depend on the strength of these synergetic support struts of precision diagnostics, tailored therapeutics, vaccine innovation, and supportive policy frameworks [108]. Efforts, particularly those such as vaccination or targeted antiviral strategies that can be coordinated across virologists, immunologists, clinicians, and public health officials will play a crucial role in minimizing disease burden and limiting impact on these individuals.

7. Conclusion

More concerning is Mpox infection in the immunocompromised. The sort of patients being considered here essentially fall under the disease category that can present atypically with more severe and devastating manifestations, prolonged viral shedding, and enormously increased risk for complications such as encephalitis, pneumonitis, secondary bacterial infections, and, under some conditions, multiorgan failure. The conditions for immunocompromise could include advanced HIV/AIDS, active cancers, extended use of immunosuppressive drugs, or some post-transplantation period. Such an immunocompromised state must not only interfere with the viral clearance but also provide an opportunity for viral dissemination in the host and again present a high-risk scenario for intercurrent infections with other opportunistic pathogens. Whenever this condition is present, early detection and diagnosis become paramount for successfully treating the disease. Such a diagnosis would include PCR detection, serological testing, viral load measurement, and cytokine profiling. Starting antiviral therapy with tecovirimat as soon as possible, alongside personalized supportive management and adjusting immunosuppressive therapy, can be life-changing. However, issues regarding these patients arise in the form of late diagnosis due to atypical presentations, poor awareness and acceptance of the Mpox vaccine among high-risk groups, and lack of existing evidence for treating those with a distinctly compromised immune system. Moving on, precision diagnostics, patient awareness, strategies for treatment based on evidence, and equity-based public health approaches must be optimized to curb Mpox-related morbidity and mortality in immunocompromised people around the globe.

Conflict of interest

None.

Author details

Maneesh Kumar[1], Pratima Gupta[1,2*], Suman Kumar[1,2*], Mithilesh Kumar Jha[2] and Ratnesh Kumar[2]

1 State Virus Research and Diagnostic Laboratory, Department of Microbiology, All India Institute of Medical Sciences, Deoghar, Jharkhand, India

2 Department of Microbiology, All India Institute of Medical Sciences, Deoghar, Jharkhand, India

*Address all correspondence to: drpratima68@gmail.com; sumankumar.kulharia@gmail.com

References

[1] Ahmed SK, Dabou EA, Ibrahim FM, Mohammed MG, Chandran D, Basit J, et al. Challenges and counteracting strategies including optimum health service practices for frontline nurses during the Mpox outbreak and futuristic vision. SAGE Open Nursing. 2024;**10**:1-10. DOI: 10:23779608241256209

[2] Martínez-Fernández DE, Fernández-Quezada D, Casillas-Muñoz FA, Carrillo-Ballesteros FJ, Ortega-Prieto AM, Jimenez-Guardeño JM, et al. Human Monkeypox: A comprehensive overview of epidemiology, pathogenesis, diagnosis, treatment, and prevention strategies. Pathogens. 2023;**12**(7):947. DOI: 10.3390/pathogens12070947

[3] Agrati C, Bartolini B, Bordoni V, Locatelli F, Capobianchi MR, Di Caro A, et al. Emerging viral infections in immunocompromised patients: A great challenge to better define the role of immune response. Frontiers in Immunology. 2023;**14**:1147871. DOI: 10.3389/fimmu.2023.1147871

[4] Cumming E, Peters C. Immune response to infection. Anaesthesia and Intensive Care Medicine. 1 Jun 2024;**25**(6):439-443. DOI: 10.1016/j.mpaic.2024.04.003

[5] Baker RE, Mahmud AS, Miller IF, Rajeev M, Rasambainarivo F, Rice BL, et al. Infectious disease in an era of global change. Nature Reviews Microbiology. 2022;**20**(4):193-205. DOI: 10.1038/s41579-021-00639-z

[6] Kim H, Kwon R, Lee H, Lee SW, Rahmati M, Koyanagi A, et al. Viral load dynamics and shedding kinetics of mpox infection: A systematic review and meta-analysis. Journal of Travel Medicine. 2023;**30**(5):taad111. DOI: 10.1093/jtm/taad111

[7] Mohanto S, Faiyazuddin M, Gholap AD, Jc D, Bhunia A, Subbaram K, et al. Addressing the resurgence of global monkeypox (Mpox) through advanced drug delivery platforms. Travel Medicine and Infectious Disease. 2023;**56**:102636. DOI: 10.1016/j.tmaid.2023.102636

[8] Titanji BK, Hazra A, Zucker J. Mpox clinical presentation, diagnostic approaches, and treatment strategies: A review. Journal of the American Medical Association. 2024;**332**(19):1652-1662. DOI: 10.1001/jama.2024.21091

[9] Reda A, Dhama K. Mpox impact on different organ systems: Complications, mechanisms, and management. Reviews in Medical Virology. 2023;**33**(4):e2443. DOI: 10.1002/rmv.2443

[10] Wang J, Goyal R, Gautam RK, Garg K, Husain S, Dubey AK, et al. Decoding and unravelling mpox, herpes, and syphilis infections: A state of art review. Current Pharmaceutical Biotechnology. 2025;**26**(10):1532-1548. DOI: 10.2174/0113892010293479240709074020

[11] Wang J, Nguyen L, Volante V, Daniel J, Preuss C. Mpox: New challenges with the disease. Rising Contagious Diseases: Basics, Management, and Treatments. 2024:20-30. DOI: 10.1002/9781394188741.ch3

[12] Gecse KB, Vermeire S. Differential diagnosis of inflammatory bowel disease: Imitations and complications. The Lancet Gastroenterology and Hepatology. 2018;**3**(9):644-653

[13] Kumar M, Kumar S, Kumar R, Jha MK, Tiwari SN, Gupta P. Azadirachta

indica natural active ingredients to cure Mpox: In silico targeting VP39. Journal of Pharmaceutical Research International. 2025;**37**(4):21-37. DOI: 10.9734/jpri/2025/v37i47676

[14] Zinnah MA, Uddin MB, Hasan T, Das S, Khatun F, Hasan MH, et al. The re-emergence of mpox: Old illness, modern challenges. Biomedicine. 2024;**12**(7):1457. DOI: 10.3390/biomedicines12071457

[15] Ugwu CL, Bragazzi NL, Wu J, Kong JD, Asgary A, Orbinski J, et al. Risk factors associated with human Mpox infection: A systematic review and meta-analysis. BMJ. Globalization and Health. 2025;**10**(2):1-14. DOI: 10.1136/bmjgh-2024-016937

[16] Gökengin D, Noori T, Alemany A, Bienkowski C, Liegon G, İnkaya AÇ, et al. Prevention strategies for sexually transmitted infections, HIV, and viral hepatitis in Europe. The Lancet Regional Health–Europe. 2023;**34**:1-16. DOI: 10.1016/j.lanepe.2023.100738

[17] Akingbola A, Adegbesan CA, Adewole O, Idahor C, Odukoya T, Nwaeze E, et al. Understanding the resurgence of mpox: Key drivers and lessons from recent outbreaks in Africa. Tropical Medicine and Health. 2025;**53**(1):1-2. DOI: 10.1186/s41182-024-00678-1

[18] Sokunbi AE, Adeyemi O. Exploring atypical manifestations of Mpox: Anarrative review. Research Journal of Health Sciences. 2024;**12**(1):71-81. DOI: 10.4314/rejhs.v12i1.9

[19] Straif-Bourgeois S, Tonzel JL, Kretzschmar M, Ratard R. Infectious disease epidemiology. In: Handbook of Epidemiology. New York, NY: Springer New York; 2023. pp. 1-79. DOI: 10.1007/978-1-4614-6625-3_34-1

[20] Khan I, Mahalakshmi S, Dixit T, Shinkre R, Ravindran S, Bandyopadhyay S, et al. Differential diagnosis, prevention measures, and therapeutic interventions for enhanced monkeypox (mpox) care. Cureus. 2024;**16**(5):e60724. DOI: 10.7759/cureus.60724

[21] Patel M, Adnan M, Aldarhami A, Bazaid AS, Saeedi NH, Alkayyal AA, et al. Current insights into diagnosis, prevention strategies, treatment, therapeutic targets, and challenges of monkeypox (Mpox) infections in human populations. Life. 2023;**13**(1):249. DOI: 10.3390/life13010249

[22] Mohapatra RK, Singh PK, Branda F, Mishra S, Kutikuppala LS, Suvvari TK, et al. Transmission dynamics, complications and mitigation strategies of the current mpox outbreak: A comprehensive review with bibliometric study. Reviews in Medical Virology. 2024;**34**(3):e2541. DOI: 10.1002/rmv.2541

[23] Selvaraj N, Shyam S, Dhurairaj P, Thiruselvan K, Thiruselvan A, Kancherla Y, et al. Mpox: Epidemiology, clinical manifestations and recent developments in treatment and prevention. Expert Review of Anti-Infective Therapy. 2023;**21**(6):641-653. DOI: 10.1080/14787210.2023.2208346

[24] Satapathy P, Khatib MN, Gaidhane S, Zahiruddin QS, Alrasheed HA, Al-Subaie MF, et al. Multi-organ clinical manifestations of Mpox: An umbrella review of systematic reviews. BMC Infectious Diseases. 2024;**24**(1):992

[25] Kumar M, Sahoo GC, Das VN, Singh K, Pandey K. A review of miRNA regulation in Japanese encephalitis (JEV) virus infection. Current Biotechnology. 2024;**25**(5):521-533. DOI: 10.2174/0113892010241606231003102047

[26] Al-Dabbagh J, Deeb EM, Younis R, Eissa R. The dermatological manifestations and differential diagnosis of monkeypox: A narrative review. Medicine. 2024;**103**(44):e40359. DOI: 10.1097/MD.0000000000040359

[27] Kumar M, Kumar R, Kumari A, Topno RK. Multiple microbial coinfections occurred during COVID-19 pandemic. IP International Journal of Medical Microbiology and Tropical Diseases. 2024b;**9**(4):209-217

[28] Chakravarty N, Hemani D, Paravastu R, Ahmad Z, Palani SN, Arumugaswami V, et al. Mpox virus and its ocular surface manifestations. The Ocular Surface. 2024;**34**:108-121. DOI: 10.1016/j.jtos.2024.07.001

[29] Simon-Gozalbo A, Gamo-Guerrero M, Alonso-Garcia S, Mauleon-Fernandez C, Cuevas-Tascon G. Haemorrhagic monkeypox infection in an immunosuppressed patient with human immunodeficiency virus: Beyond the pustules. Clinical Microbiology and Infection. 2022;**29**(1):122. DOI: 10.1016/j.cmi.2022.09.017

[30] Prabhu SR. Pathology of organ systems of the body. In: Textbook of General Pathology for Dental Students. Cham: Springer Nature Switzerland; 2023. pp. 133-146

[31] Lim EY, Jackson SE, Wills MR. The CD4+ T cell response to human cytomegalovirus in healthy and immunocompromised people. Frontiers in Cellular and Infection Microbiology. 2020;**10**:202. DOI: 10.3389/fcimb.2020.00202

[32] Protopapas K, Dimopoulou D, Kalesis N, Akinosoglou K, Moschopoulos CD. Mpox and lessons learned in the light of the recent outbreak: A narrative review. Viruses. 2024;**16**(10):1620. DOI: 10.3390/v16101620

[33] Bruno G, Buccoliero GB. Antivirals against monkeypox (Mpox) in humans: An updated narrative review. Life. 2023;**13**(10):1969. DOI: 10.3390/life13101969

[34] Raglow Z, Lauring AS. Virus evolution in prolonged infections of immunocompromised individuals. Clinical Chemistry. 2025;**71**(1):109-118. DOI: 10.1093/clinchem/hvae150

[35] Adelakun AA, Onaolapo MC, Olorunsesan MD, Oluwole F, Ajayi AF. Mpox: lessons learnt from previous viral outbreaks applicable to the ongoing outbreak: Mpox: les leçons tirées des précédentes épidémies virales applicables à l'épidémie actuelle. African Journal of Clinical and Experimental Microbiology. 2024;**25**(4):371-380. DOI: 10.4314/ajcem.v25i4.1

[36] Vouga M, Nielsen-Saines K, Dashraath P, Baud D. The monkeypox outbreak: Risks to children and pregnant women. The Lancet Child and Adolescent Health. 2022;**6**(11):751-753

[37] Ruiz-Pacheco JA, Castillo-Díaz LA, Arreola-Torres R, Fonseca-Coronado S, Gómez-Navarro B. Diabetes mellitus: Lessons from COVID-19 for monkeypox infection. Primary Care Diabetes. 2023;**17**(2):113-118. DOI: 10.1016/j.pcd.2023.01.008

[38] Grubaugh ND, Ladner JT, Lemey P, Pybus OG, Rambaut A, Holmes EC, et al. Tracking virus outbreaks in the twenty-first century. Nature Microbiology. 2019;**4**(1):10-19. DOI: 10.1038/s41564-018-0296-2

[39] Witzel TC, Ghobrial A, Palich R, Charles H, Rodger AJ, Sabin C, et al. Experiences of mpox illness and case

management among cis and trans gay, bisexual and other men who have sex with men in England: A qualitative study. EClinicalMedicine. 2024;**70**:1-11. DOI: 10.1016/j.eclinm.2024.102522

[40] da Silva SJ, Kohl A, Pena L, Pardee K. Clinical and laboratory diagnosis of monkeypox (mpox): Current status and future directions. Iscience. 2023;**26**(6):1-19. DOI: 10.1016/j.isci.2023.106759

[41] Oiwoh S, Abdullahi N, Oyakhire N, Babba Z, Umar A, Cole-Adeife O, et al. Mpox protocol by the Nigerian Association of Dermatologists: A resource for appropriate clinical and public health response. Nigerian Journal of Dermatology. 2023;**13**(3):8-29

[42] Barnes AH, Smith C, Dash A, Shishido AA. Mpox: Special considerations in the immunocompromised host. Current Treatment Options in Infectious Diseases. 2022;**14**(4):43-66

[43] Pinnetti C, Cimini E, Mazzotta V, Matusali G, Vergori A, Mondi A, et al. Mpox as AIDS-defining event with a severe and protracted course: Clinical, immunological, and virological implications. The Lancet Infectious Diseases. 2024;**24**(2):e127-e135

[44] Chaix E, Boni M, Guillier L, Bertagnoli S, Mailles A, Collignon C, et al. Risk of Monkeypox virus (MPXV) transmission through the handling and consumption of food. Microbial Risk Analysis. 2022;**22**:100237. DOI: 10.1016/j.mran.2022.100237

[45] Centers for Disease Control and Prevention. Monkeypox in the United States: What Clinicians Need to Know. 2022. Available from: https://stacks.cdc.gov>cdc>cdc_119786_DS1

[46] Aljabali AA, Obeid MA, Nusair MB, Hmedat A, Tambuwala MM. Monkeypox virus: An emerging epidemic. Microbial Pathogenesis. 2022;**173**:105794. DOI: 10.1016/j.micpath.2022.105794

[47] Ayeh MA, Cofie K, Mensah GS, Amo-Kodieh F, Kyeremeh P. Monkeypox infection: Risk assessment and clinical outcomes among immunocompromised populations in sub-Saharan Africa: A systematic review and meta-analysis. Ghana Journal of Nursing and Midwifery. 2024;**1**(4):107-124. DOI: 10.69600/gjnmid.2024.v01.i04.107-124

[48] Cordero E, Aydillo T, Farinas MC, Pano-Pardo JR, Pachon J, Viasus D, et al. Immunosuppressed patients with pandemic influenza a 2009 (H1N1) virus infection. European journal of clinical microbiology and infectious diseases. 2012;**31**:547-556

[49] Belsky JA, Tullius BP, Lamb MG, Sayegh R, Stanek JR, Auletta JJ. COVID-19 in immunocompromised patients: A systematic review of cancer, hematopoietic cell and solid organ transplant patients. Journal of Infection. 2021;**82**(3):329-338

[50] Saghazadeh A, Rezaei N. Insights on Mpox virus infection immunopathogenesis. Reviews in Medical Virology. 2023;**33**(2):e2426. DOI: 10.1002/rmv.2426

[51] Budamakuntla L, Jaidev NC, Hanumanthayya K, Eswari L, Sacchidanand S, Archana L, et al. Skin in HIV. SM Online Publishers LLC; 2015. ISBN: 978-0-9962745-2-4

[52] Dropulic LK, Lederman HM. Overview of infections in the immunocompromised host. Diagnostic Microbiology of the Immunocompromised Host. 2016:1-50. DOI: 10.1128/9781555819040.ch1

[53] Rahim K, Saleha S, Zhu X, Huo L, Basit A, Franco OL. Bacterial contribution in chronicity of wounds. Microbial Ecology. 2017;**73**:710-721. DOI: 10.1007/s00248-016-0867-9

[54] DeLeon S, Clinton A, Fowler H, Everett J, Horswill AR, Rumbaugh KP. Synergistic interactions of Pseudomonas aeruginosa and Staphylococcus aureus in an in vitro wound model. Infection and Immunity. 2014;**82**(11):4718-4728. DOI: 10.1128/IAI.02198-14

[55] Ge Y, Wang Q. Current research on fungi in chronic wounds. Frontiers in Molecular Biosciences. 2023;**9**:1057766. DOI: 10.3389/fmolb.2022.1057766

[56] Swoboda L, Held J. Impaired wound healing in diabetes. Journal of Wound Care. 2022;**31**(10):882-885. DOI: 10.12968/jowc.2022.31.10.882

[57] Azzam A, Khaled H, Salem H, Ahmed A, Heniedy AM, Hassan HS, et al. The impact of immunosuppression on the mortality and hospitalization of Monkeypox: A systematic review and meta-analysis of the 2022 outbreak. Virology Journal. 2024;**21**(1):130. DOI: 10.1186/s12985-024-02392-0

[58] Barbhuiya PA, Laskar MA, Talukdar S, Kumari P, Pathak MP. Current trends in diagnostics, biomarker identification, and drug discovery targeting Monkeypox (Mpox). The Microbe. 2025;7:100330. DOI: 10.1016/j.microb.2025.100330

[59] Sharma E, Malhotra S, Kaul S, Jain N, Nagaich U. Unveiling the Mpox menace: Exploring the intricacies of a zoonotic virus and clinical implications. Diagnostic Microbiology and Infectious Disease. 2023;**107**(2):116024

[60] Alalawi F, Alhadari F, Tobia H, Alhadari A. Monkeypox in a kidney transplant recipient: Case report and literature review. Experimental and Clinical Transplantation. 2023;**21**:913-916. DOI: 10.6002/ect.2023.0222

[61] Taha AM, Elrosasy A, Mahmoud AM, Saed SA, Moawad WA, Hamouda E, et al. The effect of HIV and mpox co-infection on clinical outcomes: Systematic review and meta-analysis. HIV Medicine. 2024;**25**(8):897-909

[62] Saldana CS, Kelley CF, Aldred BM, Cantos VD. Mpox and HIV: A narrative review. Current HIV/AIDS Reports. 2023;**20**(4):261-269

[63] Bogacka A, Wroczynska A, Rymer W, Grzesiowski P, Kant R, Grzybek M, et al. MPOX unveiled: Global epidemiology, treatment advances, and prevention strategies. One Health. 2025;**20**:101030. DOI: 10.1016/j.onehlt.2025.101030

[64] Schuch A, Hoh A, Thimme R. The role of natural killer cells and CD8+ T cells in hepatitis B virus infection. Frontiers in Immunology. 2014;**5**:258

[65] Bekker LG, Beyrer C, Mgodi N, Lewin SR, Delany-Moretlwe S, Taiwo B, et al. HIV infection. Nature Reviews Disease Primers. 2023;**9**(1):42

[66] Adamo S, Gao Y, Sekine T, Mily A, Wu J, Storgärd E, et al. Memory profiles distinguish cross-reactive and virus-specific T cell immunity to mpox. Cell Host and Microbe. 2023;**31**(6):928-936

[67] Azari PP, Rukerd MR, Charostad J, Bashash D, Farsiu N, Behzadi S, et al. Innate immune responses: Insights into evasion mechanisms and potential therapeutic strategies. Cytokine. 2024;**183**:156751

[68] Hickman HD, Moutsopoulos NM. Viral infection and antiviral immunity in the oral cavity. Nature Reviews

Immunology. 2024;**25**:235-249. DOI: 10.1038/s41577-024-01100-x

[69] Harbour JC, Abdelbary M, Schell JB, Fancher SP, McLean JJ, Nappi TJ, et al. T helper 1 effector memory CD4+ T cells protect the skin from poxvirus infection. Cell Reports. 2023;**42**(5):112407. DOI: 10.1016/j.celrep.2023.112407

[70] Acharya A, Kumar N, Singh K, Byrareddy SN. Mpox in MSM: Tackling stigma, minimizing risk factors, exploring pathogenesis, and treatment approaches. Biomedical Journal. 2024;**48**(1):100746. DOI: 10.1016/j.bj.2024.100746

[71] Liu BM, Rakhmanina NY, Yang Z, Bukrinsky MI. Mpox (Monkeypox) virus and its co-infection with HIV, sexually transmitted infections, or bacterial superinfections: Double whammy or a new prime culprit? Viruses. 2024;**16**(5):784. DOI: 10.3390/v16050784

[72] Hussain MS, Gupta G, Samuel VP, Almalki WH, Kazmi I, Alzarea SI, et al. Immunopathology of herpes simplex virus-associated neuroinflammation: Unveiling the mysteries. Reviews in Medical Virology. 2024;**34**(1):e2491

[73] Anil S, Joseph B, Thomas M, Sweety VK, Suresh N, Waltimo T. Monkeypox: A viral zoonotic disease of rising global concern. Infectious Diseases and Immunity. 2024;**4**(03):121-131

[74] Kumar S, Guruparan D, Karuppanan K, Kumar KS. Comprehensive insights into Monkeypox (mpox): Recent advances in epidemiology, diagnostic approaches and therapeutic strategies. Pathogens. 2024;**14**(1):1

[75] Adelino TÉ, Santos SC, Lima MT, da Costa AV, Guimarães NR, Tomé LM, et al. Differential diagnosis of exanthematous viruses during the 2022 Mpox outbreak in Minas Gerais, Brazil. Journal of Clinical Microbiology. 2024;**62**(6):e00103-e00124

[76] Branda F, Romano C, Ciccozzi M, Giovanetti M, Scarpa F, Ciccozzi A, et al. Mpox: An overview of pathogenesis, diagnosis, and public health implications. Journal of Clinical Medicine. 2024;**13**(8):2234

[77] Stingone C, Sarmati L, Andreoni M. The clinical Spectrum of human immunodeficiency virus infection. Sexually Transmitted Infections: Advances in Understanding and Management. 2020:295-317. DOI: 10.1007/978-3-030-02200-6_15

[78] Pourkarim F, Entezari-Maleki T. Clinical considerations on monkeypox antiviral medications: An overview. Pharmacology Research and Perspectives. 2024;**12**(1):e01164. DOI: 10.1002/prp2.1164

[79] Agrawal A, Ison MG, Danziger-Isakov L. Long-term infectious complications of kidney transplantation. Clinical Journal of the American Society of Nephrology. 2022;**17**(2):286-295. DOI: 10.2215/CJN.15971020

[80] Rao AK. Interim clinical treatment considerations for severe manifestations of mpox—United States, February 2023. MMWR. Morbidity and Mortality Weekly Report. 2023;**72**:232-243. DOI: 10.15585/mmwr.mm7209a4

[81] Alhumaid S, Al Mutair A, Al Alawi Z, Alshawi AM, Alomran SA, Almuhanna MS, et al. Coinfections with bacteria, fungi, and respiratory viruses in patients with SARS-CoV-2: A systematic review and meta-analysis. Pathogens. 2021;**10**(7):809. DOI: 10.3390/pathogens10070809

[82] Rider P, Carmi Y, Cohen I. Biologics for targeting inflammatory

cytokines, clinical uses, and limitations. International Journal of Cell Biology. 2016;**2016**(1):9259646

[83] Hazra A, Cherabie JN. Is mpox a sexually transmitted infection? Why narrowing the scope of this disease may be harmful. Clinical Infectious Diseases. 2023;**76**(8):1504-1507. DOI: 10.1093/cid/ciac962

[84] Linfield RY, Nguyen NN, Laprade OH, Holodniy M, Chary A. An update on drug–drug interactions in older adults living with human immunodeficiency virus (HIV). Expert Review of Clinical Pharmacology. 2024;**17**(7):589-614. DOI: 10.1080/17512433.2024.2350968

[85] Sahin TK, Kaygusuz Y, İcli MC, Aksoy S, Guven DC. The perspectives and knowledge of patients with cancer on mpox and mpox vaccination: A cross-sectional study. Current Medical Research and Opinion. 2025;**41**(1):83-91. DOI: 10.1080/03007995.2024.2445757

[86] Aggarwal S, Agarwal P, Nigam K, Vijay N, Yadav P, Gupta N. Mapping the landscape of health research priorities for effective pandemic preparedness in human mpox virus disease. Pathogens. 2023;**12**(11):1352. DOI: 10.3390/pathogens12111352

[87] Temsah MH, Aljamaan F, Alenezi S, Abouammoh N, Alhasan K, Dasuqi SA, et al. Monkeypox disease (MPOX) perceptions among healthcare workers versus general population during the first month of the WHO alert: Cross-sectional survey in Saudi Arabia. Vaccine. 2022;**10**(12):2071

[88] Halahleh K, Arai Y, Gavriilaki E. Post-transplant complications. Blood Cell Therapy. 2023;**6**(1):23. DOI: 10.31547/bct-2022-021

[89] Heald-Sargent T, Michaels MG, Ardura MI. Pre-transplantation strategies for infectious disease mitigation and prevention. Journal of the Pediatric Infectious Diseases Society. 2024;**13**(Suppl. 1):S3-S13. DOI: 10.1093/jpids/piad075

[90] Suliman O, Joomye M, Wu HH, Chinnadurai R. Monkeypox infection in kidney transplant recipients. Clinical Kidney Journal. 2025;**18**(3):sfaf048. DOI: 10.1093/ckj/sfaf048/8010847

[91] Higgins E, Ranganath N, Mehkri O, Majeed A, Walker J, Spivack S, et al. Clinical features, treatment, and outcomes of mpox in solid organ transplant recipients: A multicenter case series and literature review. American Journal of Transplantation. 2023;**23**(12):1972-1979. DOI: 10.1016/j.ajt.2023.07.016

[92] Rana S, Joshi V, Sahoo GC, Kumar M, Pandey K. Upsurge in antibiotic-resistant infections. In: Emerging Paradigms for Antibiotic-Resistant Infections: Beyond the Pill. Singapore: Springer Nature Singapore; 2024. pp. 25-42. DOI: 10.1007/978-981-97-5272-0_2

[93] Ritter JM, Martines RB, Bhatnagar J, Rao AK, Villalba JA, Silva-Flannery L, et al. Pathology and Monkeypox virus localization in tissues from immunocompromised patients with severe or fatal mpox. The Journal of Infectious Diseases. 2024;**229**(Suppl. 2):S219-S228. DOI: 10.1093/infdis/jiad574

[94] McKean J, Ronan-Bentle S. Abdominal pain in the immunocompromised patient—Human immunodeficiency virus, transplant, cancer. Emergency Medicine Clinics. 2016;**34**(2):377-386

[95] Bathina A, Kollipara H, Sravani G, Laxmi VS. Beyond classic leprosy: Exploring atypical manifestations and their diagnostic challenges. Cureus. 2024;**16**(12):e75957. DOI: 10.7759/cureus.75957

[96] Shafaati M, Zandi M. Monkeypox virus neurological manifestations in comparison to other orthopoxviruses. Travel Medicine and Infectious Disease. 2022;**49**:102414

[97] Hetta HF, Alharbi AA, Alsharif SM, Alkindy TT, Alkhamali A, Albalawi AS, et al. Mpox virus infection and vaccination: Immunopathogenesis and exploring the link to neuropsychiatric manifestations. Immuno. 2024;**4**(4):578-600

[98] Deb S, Mondal R, Sen P, Chowdhury D, Sarkar S, Banerjee G, et al. Neuroinflammatory disorders of the central nervous system associated with monkeypox virus: A systematic review and call to action. BMC Medicine. 2025;**23**:86. DOI: 10.1186/s12916-025-03921-6

[99] Bahakel H, Feldman AG, Danziger-Isakov L. Immunization of solid organ transplant candidates and recipients: A 2022 update. Infectious Disease Clinics. 2023;**37**(3):427-441. DOI: 10.1016/j.idc.2023.03.004

[100] Zhou Y, Chen Z. Mpox: A review of laboratory detection techniques. Archives of Virology. 2023;**168**(8):221. DOI: 10.1007/s00705-023-05848-w

[101] Chauhan RP, Fogel R, Limson J. Overview of diagnostic methods, disease prevalence and transmission of MPOX (formerly monkeypox) in humans and animal reservoirs. Microorganisms. 2023;**11**(5):1186. DOI: 10.3390/microorganisms11051186

[102] Siegrist EA, Sassine J. Antivirals with activity against mpox: A clinically oriented review. Clinical Infectious Diseases. 2023;**76**(1):155-164

[103] Scholz EM, Kashuba AD. The lymph node reservoir: Physiology, HIV infection, and antiretroviral therapy. Clinical Pharmacology and Therapeutics. 2021;**109**(4):918-927. DOI: 10.1002/cpt.2186

[104] Patel M, Surti M, Adnan M. Artificial intelligence (AI) in monkeypox infection prevention. Journal of Biomolecular Structure and Dynamics. 2023;**41**(17):8629-8633

[105] Gupta AK, Talukder M, Rosen T, Piguet V. Differential diagnosis, prevention, and treatment of mpox (monkeypox): A review for dermatologists. American Journal of Clinical Dermatology. 2023;**24**(4):541-556

[106] Kamei K. Live attenuated vaccines in patients receiving immunosuppressive agents. Pediatric Nephrology. 2023;**38**(12):3889-3900. DOI: 10.1007/s00467-023-05969-z

[107] Duarte PM, Adesola RO, Priyadarsini S, Singh R, Shaheen MN, Ogundijo OA, et al. Unveiling the global surge of Mpox (Monkeypox): A comprehensive review of current evidence. The Microbe. 2024;**4**:100141. DOI: 10.1016/j.microb.2024.100141

[108] Ahmed SK, Mohamed MG, Dabou EA, Abuijlan I, Chandran D, El-Shall NA, et al. Monkeypox (mpox) in immunosuppressed patients. F1000Research. 2023;**12**:127. DOI: 10.12688/f1000research.130272.2